Table of Contents

I0448108

get your free permaculture checklist now @
regenerative.com/book-checklist

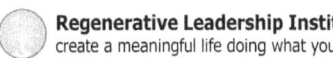

Regenerative Leadership Institute
create a meaningful life doing what you love

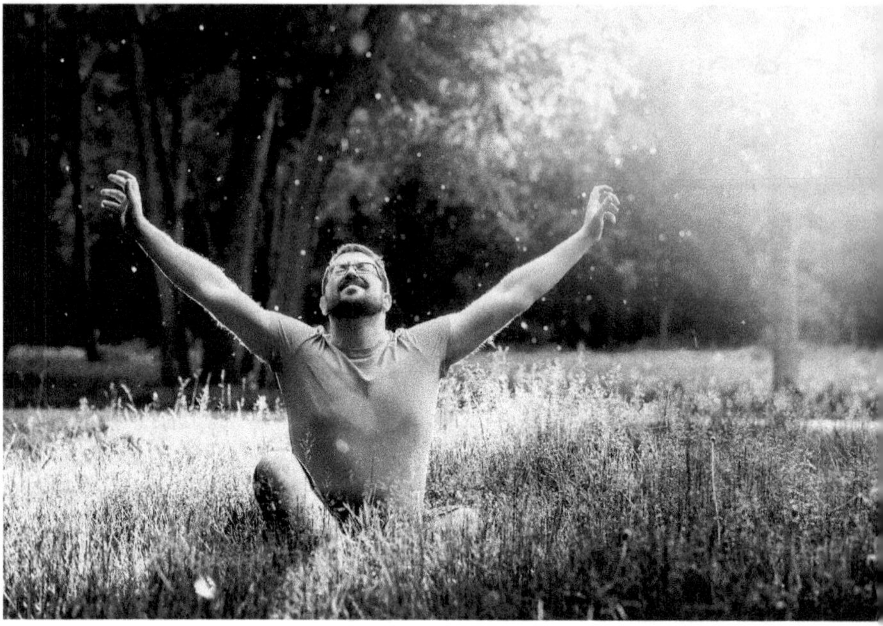

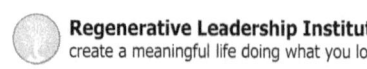

Waking Up

"Take care of your body. It's the only place you have to live."

Jim Rohn, author and motivational speaker on personal development

It happens to all of us. One day, we wake up and find that we want more for ourselves. More zest for life. Another taste of that invincibility many of us experience as young children. A greater sense of well-being.

Sometimes this happens when we're at the top of our game: you become eager to reach the next rung on the ladder once you have mastered the level you stand on now. Perhaps you've landed on a set of routines – balanced diet, regular exercise, and so on – that feels good and fine, but you wonder what it is like to feel *great*. Maybe you became curious about what it must feel like to be even healthier, lighter, more energetic and invigorated. Perhaps your habits up until

Regenerative Leadership Institute
create a meaningful life doing what you love

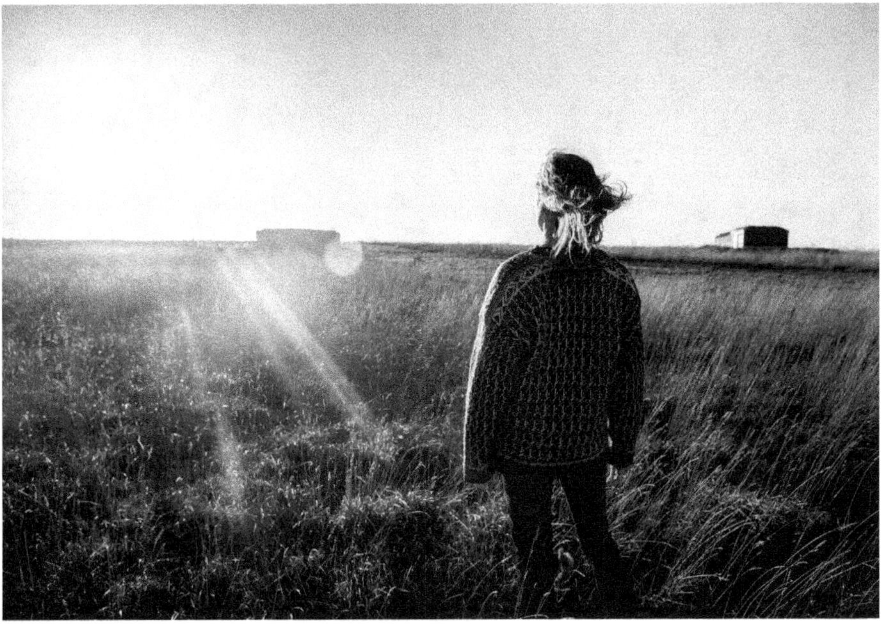

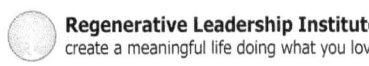

now are sufficient, but you wonder how much better you could feel if they were *optimal*.

Somewhere inside, you know it will take a little more of *something* to do that. Maybe that's how you found yourself here: you're looking to unlock your *something more*.

Or, maybe you simply want to do everything possible to lock down the odds in your favor that you'll be around to see the people you love celebrate milestones in their lives: births, graduations, weddings. Perhaps you want to not only live long but also live *well*, thriving into old age.

Or, possibly dissatisfaction with something prompted you to reflect and envision something different and better for yourself. Maybe you caught a glimpse of yourself in the gym mirror and didn't love what you saw, or maybe you find yourself fantasizing what it would be like to have more energy to keep up with your life. Maybe you have been prescribed more

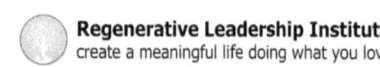

medications than you can count for chronic conditions, and you wonder if there is a better way to manage and improve your health. Maybe you are frustrated by frequent unpleasant symptoms, poor sleep, chronic pain, or unsuccessful attempts to lose weight, and you are eager to learn more about what you can do to further help yourself.

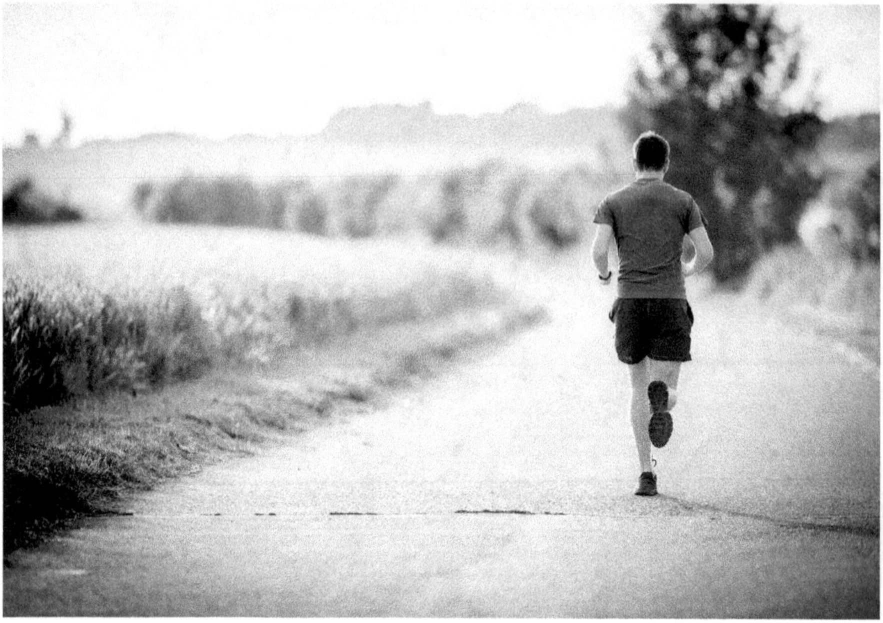

For still some others, the situation is urgent. Obesity, type 2 diabetes, cardiovascular disease, high cholesterol, and high blood pressure are all mounting a widespread blitz on the health of millions of us. Perhaps you are among those whose doctor presses you to eat and/or live differently so you can steer clear of the consequences of significant threats to your health.

Regardless of how you got here, you are ready for any or all of these:
• More vitality and vigor
• Less chronic pain and other symptoms
• Fewer mood swings and energy crashes

Regenerative Leadership Institute
create a meaningful life doing what you love

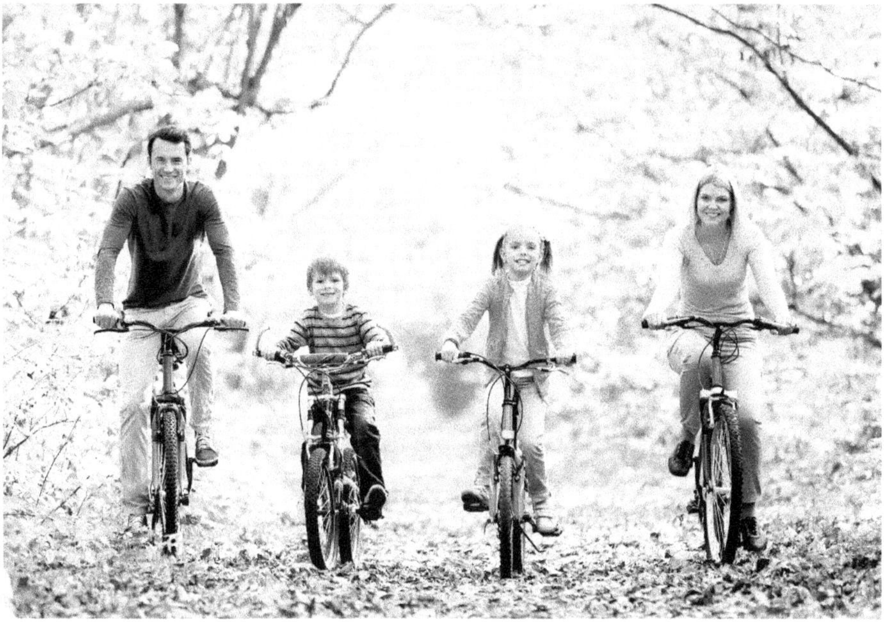

- Natural and sustainable weight loss
- Better health numbers
- Optimal health and well-being!

No matter your starting point, you have surely noticed a special glow and energy in certain people. It probably made you curious to explore how to get more of that in your own life.

Maybe you even caught a glimpse of it yourself as the euphoria following a gratifying exercise session or game of your favorite sport, or the clarity and buzz during a rejuvenating vacation or juice cleanse, or the high following a deeply satisfying moment with a loved one.

Is it possible to feel like that more of the time?

Watching these people, it is as if they have stumbled upon a secret key that unlocks the door to radiant skin, bright eyes, calm self-assurance,

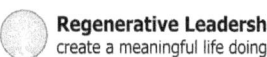

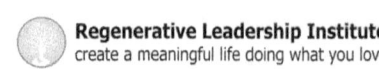

and lasting vitality. You wonder what they must do to feel so, so good every day.

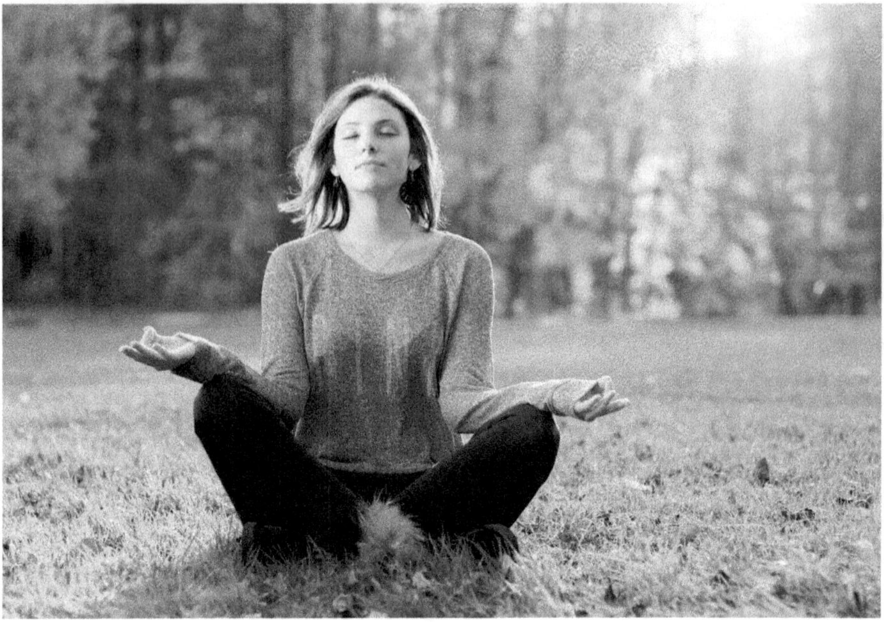

What do they eat for dinner? What do they snack on? Do they have to exercise or meditate for half the day in order to be so energetic and serene? How do they seem to thrive without a constant influx of sugary drinks and pastries to make it through the day?

You're about to find out! No matter your starting point, you are in the right place.*1

The truth is that you need not exercise or meditate to achieve a greater sense of well-being and vitality. You simply need to bring more

1 *Note: This Book primarily features sustainable weight loss and healthy lifestyle change. We will assume that you want to lose weight as part of your journey to a healthier you, but what we don't assume is how much you want to lose, or why. The challenges and solutions discussed here will help you naturally arrive at or maintain a healthy weight for your body. Therefore, this approach will support you whether you want to lose weight, increase your overall energy and health without the weight loss, or both.*

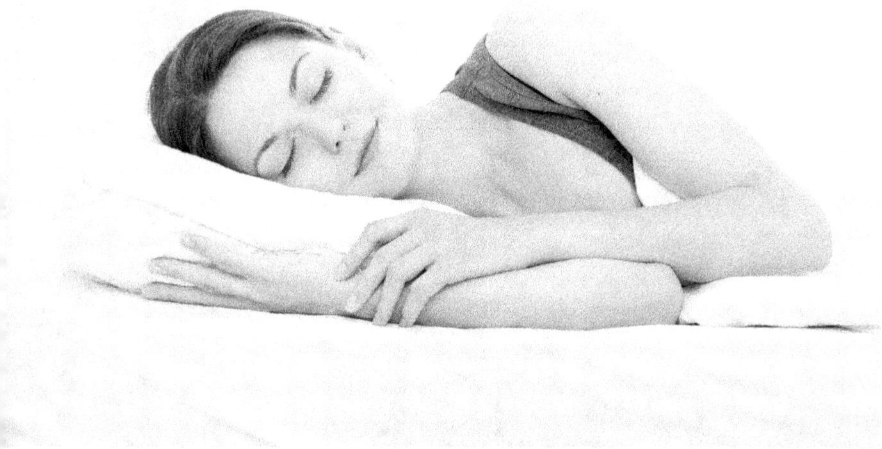

awareness to what you feed your body and mind. You may be pretty aware already, or you may realize you have never given much thought to your eating habits up until now.

Either way, what is true for everyone is that our eating and lifestyle habits have a huge impact on our mood, energy level, quality of sleep, digestion, and management or prevention of chronic diseases and other recurring symptoms. If you struggle with bothersome cravings, frequent bouts of sluggishness, recurring nasal congestion or constipation or other physical discomfort, your food may have something to do with it. If your energy and ability to concentrate feel inconsistent, if you would like to have more control over your mood swings or sudden hunger pangs, this book will show you how easy it is to make gradual changes to your eating habits that put you back in the driver's seat with greater control over your energy, mood, and satiety.

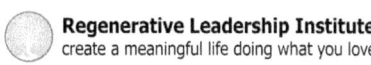

Regenerative Leadership Institute
create a meaningful life doing what you love

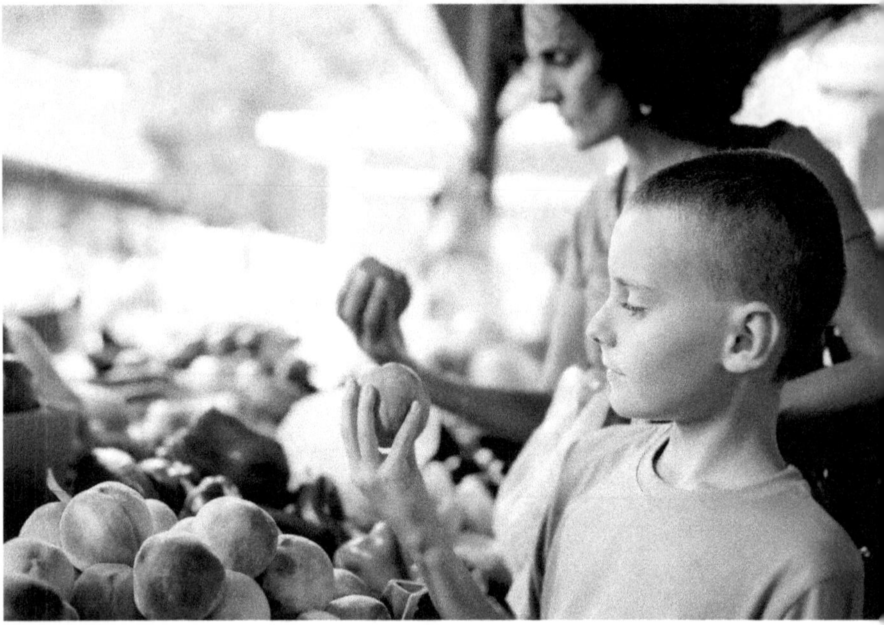

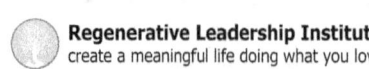

In as little as a couple weeks, for some even sooner, you will notice differences in how you look and feel after trying out our healthful eating and lifestyle plan for yourself.

How We Got Here

"We are a nation of food addicts, not metaphorically but literally. Americans eat 146 pounds of sugar and 152 pounds of flour every year. That's almost a pound of sugar and flour for every man, woman, and child in America every single day! It has led to an epidemic of unprecedented obesity and disease."

Mark Hyman, MD, functional medicine physician and best-selling author of several books including *The Blood Sugar Solution*

If you are like most Americans, you might feel run-down most of the time, restricted by general discomfort or chronic symptoms, or find yourself overweight by a little or a lot. You may wonder how you got

Regenerative Leadership Institute
create a meaningful life doing what you love

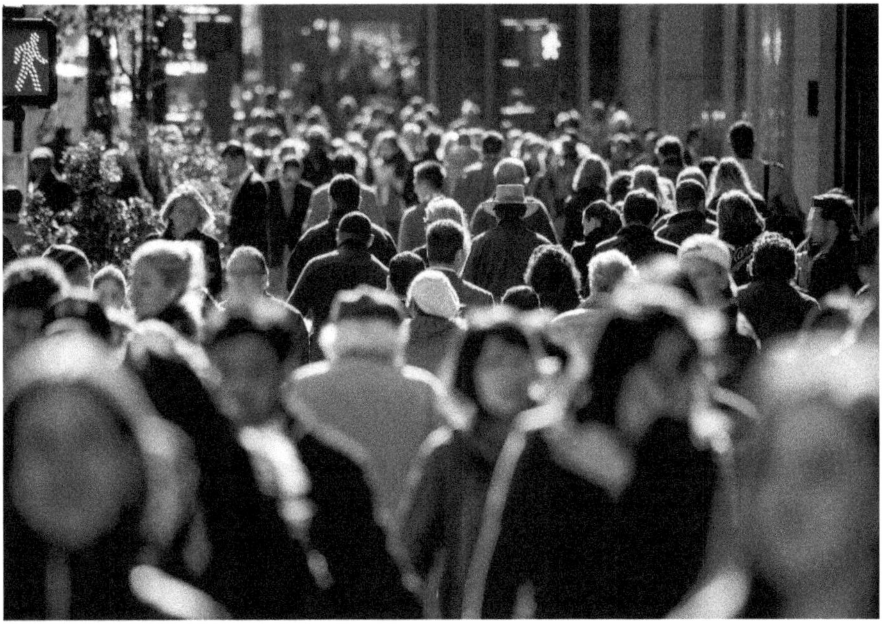

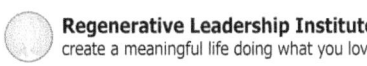

here. Some people write it off as an unavoidable accompaniment to aging. They are inevitable side effects of graduating from the teenage years to adulthood, or from younger adult to mid-life or older adulthood, right? Simple changes to our grocery store list or daily lunch order at the café surely can't make that much of a difference ... or can they?

The fact is that more and more of us find ourselves feeling run-down in some way or another while we are still quite young, even. What explains this?

While we no longer have to outrun saber tooth tigers, life is increasingly demanding in other ways. Our attention is pulled in more directions than we even realize. After you walk the dog, work a full day and perhaps answer work-related emails and calls on your off-hours, pick up the kids if you have them, worry about or pay the bills, survive a commute on jam-packed freeways or public transit... who has time or energy left to take exquisite care of themselves?

Regenerative Leadership Institute
create a meaningful life doing what you love

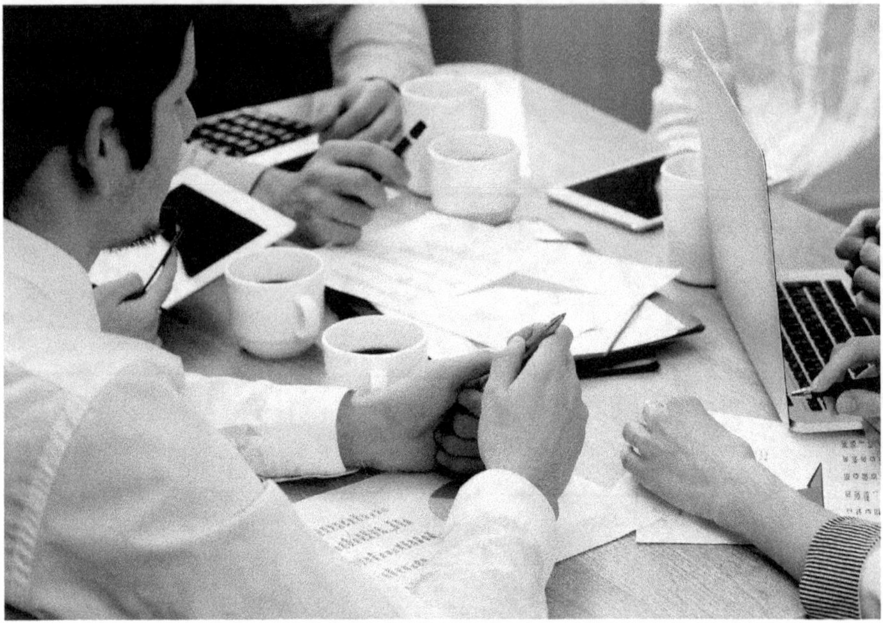

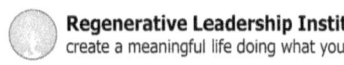

What's more, we are confronted with over 200 food and beverage-related decisions every day whether we realize it or not, and this drains our finite energy and attention. Food is more accessible than ever, and our culture encourages us to eat anytime, anywhere, whether it's mealtime or not, whether we are hungry or not. The high-calorie, high-sugar, and high-sodium packaged snacks are often the easiest to find in our office building's vending machine, the corner store, or the local café.

Our workplaces, the environment where we easily spend the majority of our waking hours, are rarely supportive of self-care practices and other healthy eating habits. The workplace culture in some businesses is changing with the growing popularity of workplace wellness programs, but still too many of us work in a job that requires us to remain seated, eyes glued to an electronic screen, and work long hours. Caffeine, soda and other sugary sweetened drinks, and high-sugar snacks and desserts usually dominate the vending machines, cafeterias or snack shops in or near our workplace, and its convenience understandably wins out.

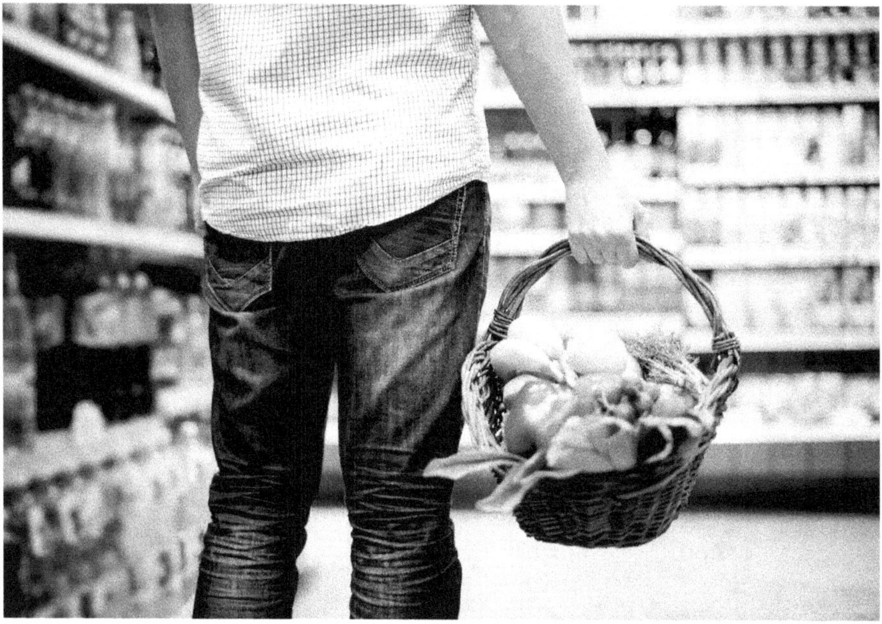

It can be really hard to set and stick to our priorities, even those about our health.

But there is a way to revitalize your health and well-being – and it is easier than you think. Remember that glow and radiance we mentioned? You're about to find out just what it takes to get there.

All it takes is your willingness to explore and experiment to find what uniquely works for you and your body. All it takes is realizing that the quality of your food has real consequences for both our day-to-day vitality as well as long-term disease prevention and management. That glow and radiance come naturally when you eat as close to the source as possible – whole, plant-based foods, as fresh and minimally processed as possible, brimming with vitamins, minerals and other

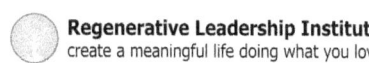

Regenerative Leadership Institute
create a meaningful life doing what you love

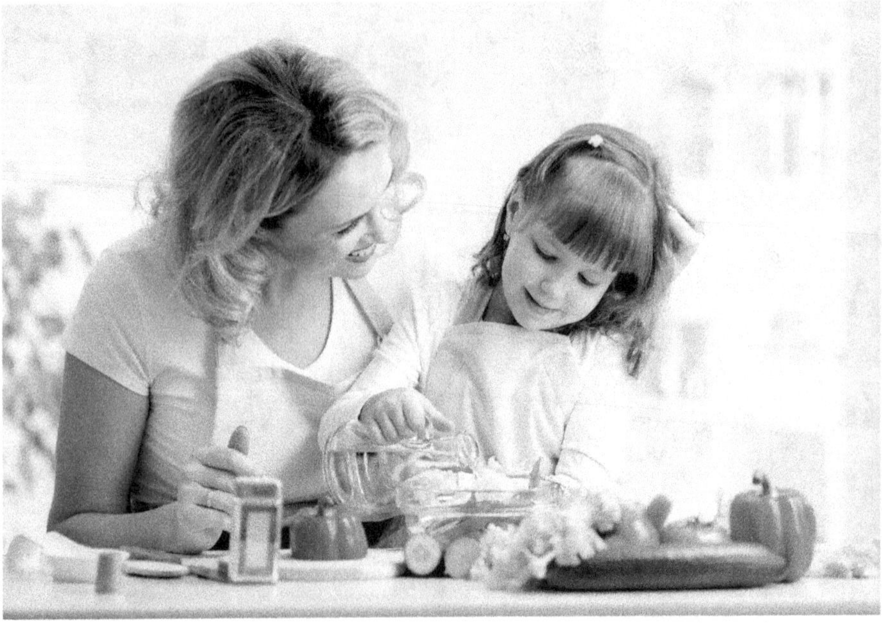

nutrients unique to plant-based foods that do wonders for our health. At every meal, each snack, you have a choice, and you will soon find that making more choices from the world of whole, plant-based foods leaves you feeling more energetic, healthier, and lighter than ever.

But first, let's discuss our current food environment. What does the average American diet currently look like? Where is there room for improvement, and why is it so important that we make those improvements? If you follow the average American diet, too, how can you benefit from a new way of eating?

The Standard American Diet, or S.A.D.

Depleted by demanding and stressful lifestyles, many of us find ourselves faced with the task – and it may even feel like a chore – of filling our fuel tank. Yep, it's time to eat.

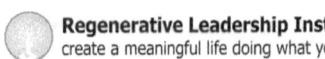

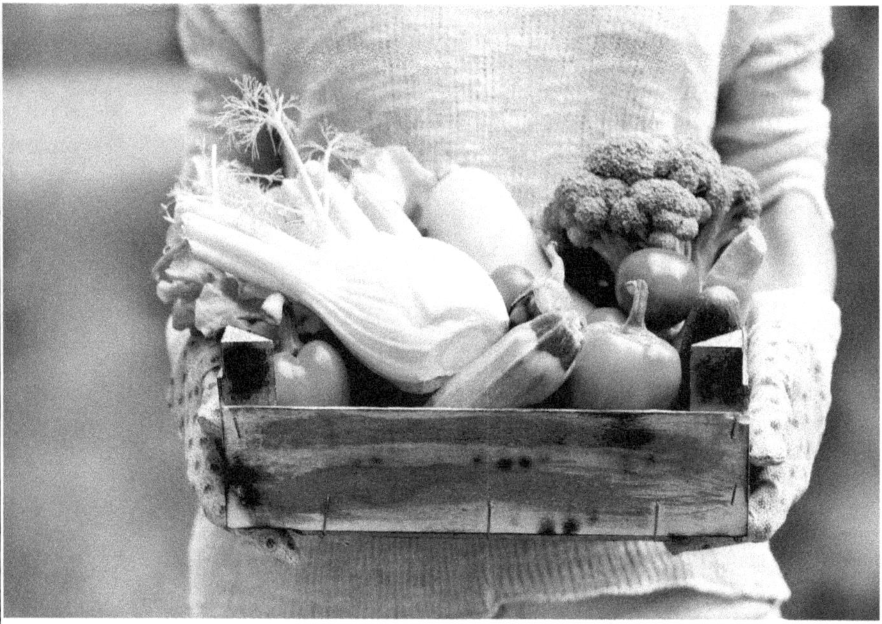

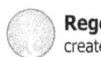

The Standard American Diet, sometimes called S.A.D., encompasses our contemporary food environment. The S.A.D. often features calorically dense foods that offer little nutrition (think vitamins, minerals, and other key nutrients) in return. This way of eating is known for its bagels, muffins and cookies, burgers, side dishes like French fries or dinner rolls, multi-layer sandwiches with generous portions of highly processed and salted meats and cheeses, sweetened and caffeinated beverages from soda to mocha to energy drinks, and frozen pizzas and pastas. Vegetables and fruit are more often seen as garnishes and side dishes, less often as the main attraction, more often making their way to our plates after canning or underneath high-calorie, high-sugar dressings and sauces, less often in their fresh and unadulterated form. If the way we feed our children is any reflection of our national food culture, recall the recent controversy in the funding and governing of our national school lunch program that concluded that ketchup on French fries and tomato paste on pizza do in fact count as a serving of vegetables.

Regenerative Leadership Institute
create a meaningful life doing what you love

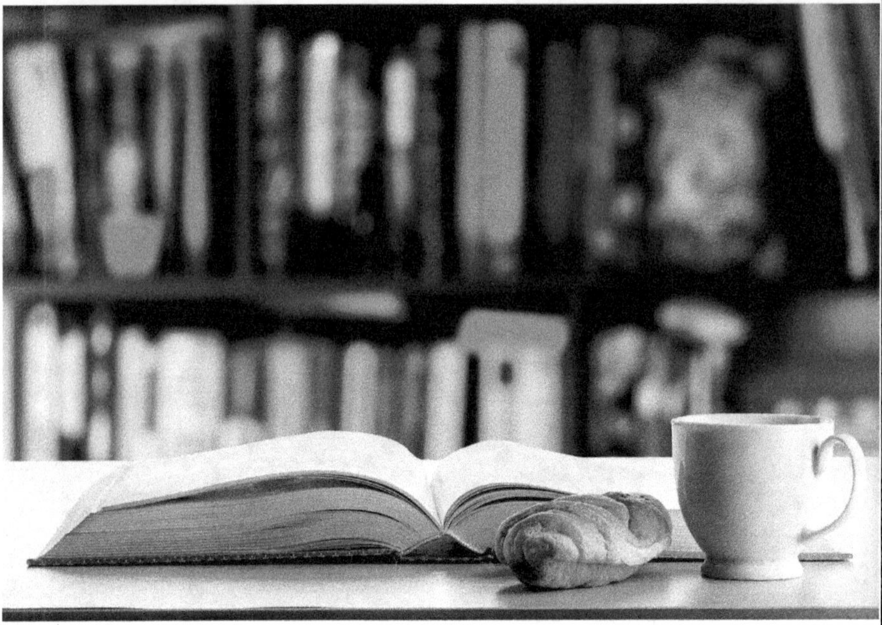

Visit the average American grocery store's snack aisle, and the average snack product is high in refined flours and sugars – corn syrup and white flour are the main, if not only, ingredients in the pastries and other baked goods, chips and crackers, snack bars, and candy and cookies that take over this aisle. As you will see in the next sections, this reliance on refined flours, refined sugars, and overall high intake of sugar, salt, and unhealthy fats lead to poor blood sugar management and sluggish metabolism in the short term, affecting many aspects of our daily life from sleep quality to energy to mood. The long-term effects of the S.A.D. are also discouraging, as evidenced by the ballooning rates of heart disease, high cholesterol, type 2 diabetes, and other chronic conditions all around us.

No longer hunting and gathering for our daily bread, we now enjoy 24/7 access to food as never before. Remember when all you could buy at a gas station was gas? Or, when the only thing available at a bookstore was, well, books? Now, locations like these are any-time-of-day opportunities to eat. Gas stations come complete with mini-marts,

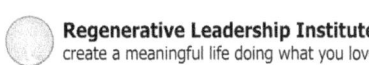

and no bookstore is complete without a cute café offering fancy coffee drinks and pastries galore.

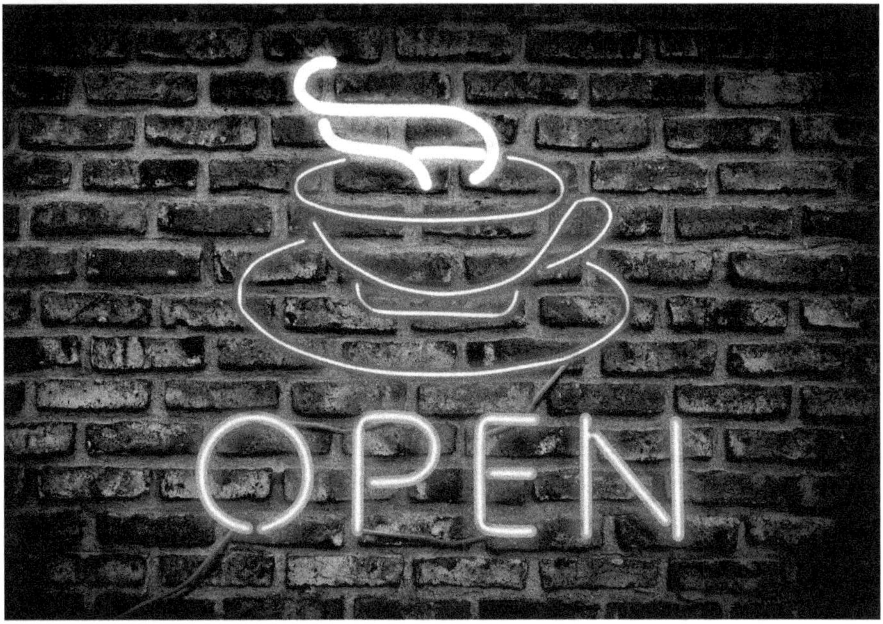

Whether it is mealtime or not, whether we feel genuine hunger in the given moment or not, this is hardly the point. Implicit messages reach our conscious and subconscious awareness on a daily basis through printed billboards, food industry commercials on radio and TV, magazine ads, restaurants and coffee shops open at all hours. We are encouraged to grab a bite here, sip on a sweetened coffee drink or soda there, treat yourself to something after a hard day, nibble on refreshments during business meetings or other events, slip into a drive-thru for a quick snack, and so on, whether we act on these messages or not.

Even our cars reflect our food environment: remember when cars came without drink holders inside? The auto industry knows we eat in our cars, and they had to respond to that. In Michael Pollan's 2008 *In Defense of Food*, he indicated that we eat about 20% of meals in our cars.

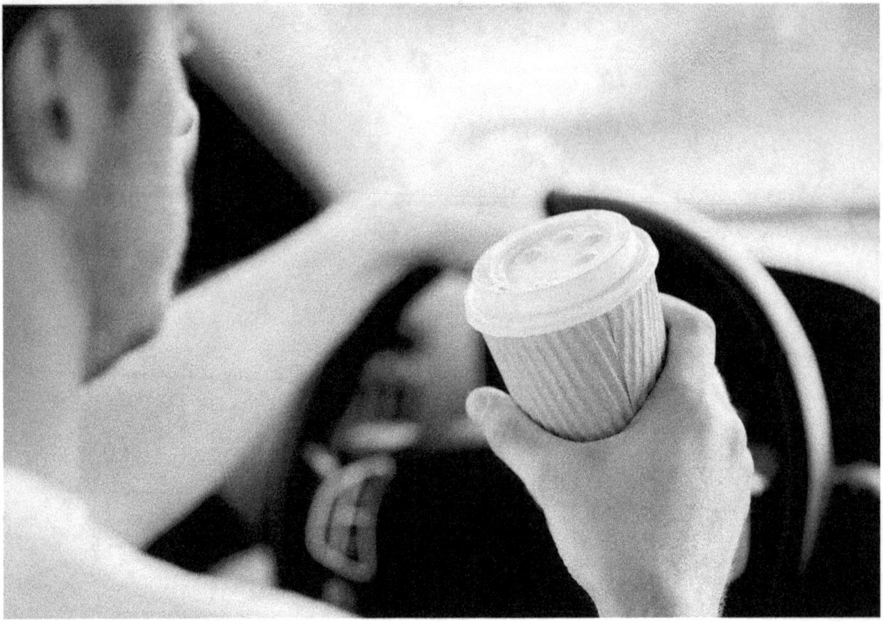

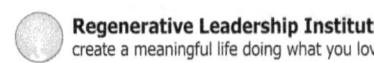

At three meals a day, seven days a week, that comes to more than 4 meals a week completely on the go and on the road. That's astounding!

Increasingly, "food products" dominate today's food environment. In contrast to whole foods, which are relatively unchanged from their original state in nature, food products are highly processed with high levels of sugar, fat, and salt, all designed and engineered to generate cravings. Packaged and processed food products trigger both blood sugar spikes and blood sugar crashes, creating a vicious cycle of mood and energy swings often accompanied by bothersome cravings. Food products are cheap, easy to overeat, high on calories, low on vitamins and minerals, and quite convenient.

Consequences

Unfortunately, this way of eating has consequences that are far less convenient. Since lifestyle and diet are the most influential

Regenerative Leadership Institute
create a meaningful life doing what you love

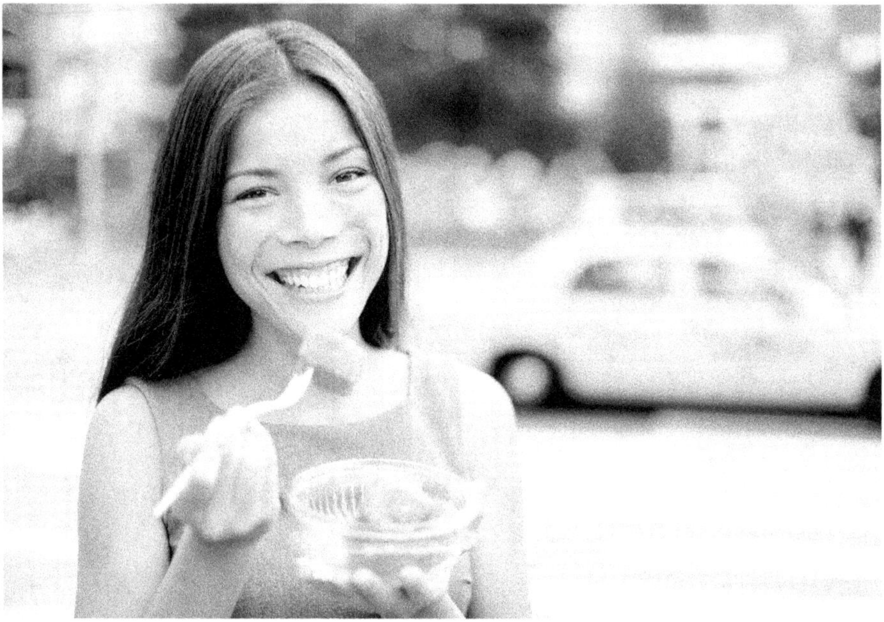

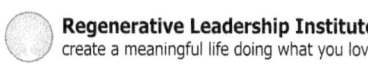

determinants of health, the Standard American Diet combined with the high-stress and hectic lifestyle that most of us experience is a recipe for disaster. ***There is a better way, and it comes down to two words: nutrient density.***

These food products are low nutrient-density foods. Meaning, an engineered, packaged food product has fewer nutrients per calorie (especially vitamins, minerals, and phytonutrients) than just about any whole food. Typically, they are not very satiating, or, satisfying. So, we eat, and eat, and eat.

Eating the S.A.D. is a major contributor to the development of Metabolic Disorder. This is the cluster of maladies that includes type 2 diabetes, obesity, cardiovascular disease, high cholesterol, and high blood pressure. It's often said: genetics is the gun, environment loads the gun, but behavior pulls the trigger. More than ever, as a nation, we rely on over-the-counter and prescription medications to

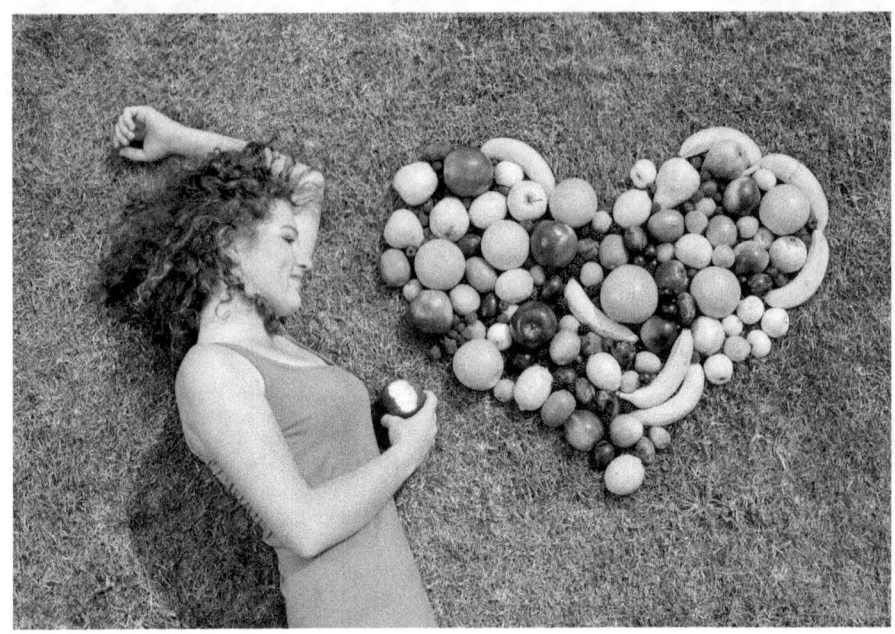

manage these and other illnesses with roots in our lifestyles and diets. Ultimately, even if it does not jeopardize your health today, the S.A.D. still robs you of the optimal energy that could be yours to fuel even more vitality and well-being.

Fortunately, the opportunity to change your fate comes about three times a day, if not more! Better blood sugar control and insulin response, interruption or reversal of conditions like heart disease and high blood pressure, improvement of other key health numbers linked to longevity and quality of life – a very strong case is emerging from years of research that our eating and lifestyle habits have more to do with these chronic conditions than we previously thought. Simple changes, substitutions and swaps in your daily diet have been shown to improve health numbers in a matter of weeks and months, and we are here to show you the way!

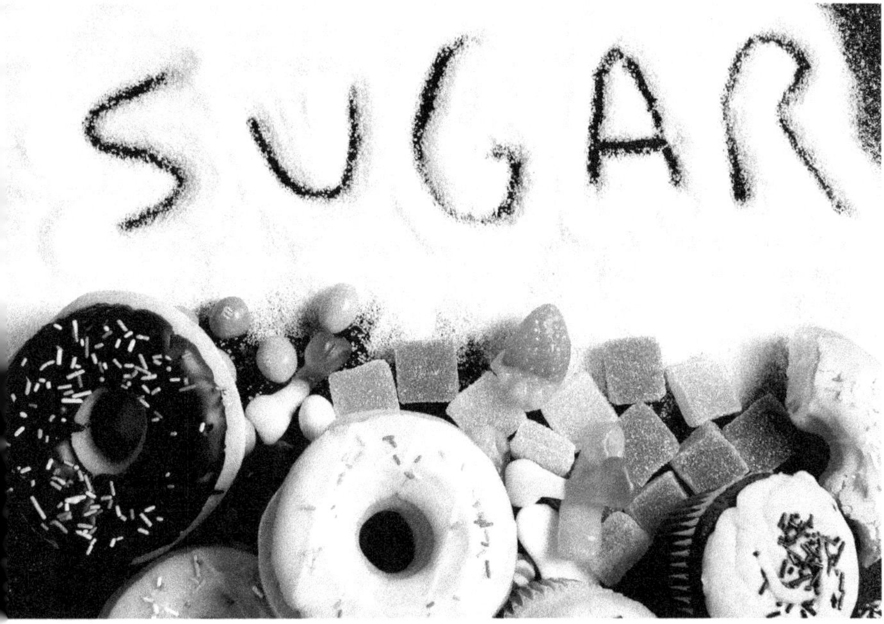

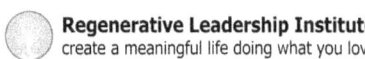

Sugar: A Special Case

"My advice is to give up stevia, aspartame, sucralose, sugar alcohols like xylitol and malitol, and all of the other heavily used and marketed sweeteners unless you want to slow down your metabolism, gain weight, and become an addict."

Mark Hyman, MD, functional medicine physician and best-selling author of several books including *The Blood Sugar Solution*

Sugar deserves a special warning label all of its own because of its pervasive presence in our food supply and its unique appeal to our tastebuds and biological reward systems. Moderation in all things, sure, but there really ought to be an exception for sugar.

Here's why: research supports the notion that consumption of refined and added sugars triggers cravings that are stronger than those elicited by cocaine. Yes, cocaine. This may sound overdramatic or extreme,

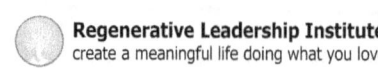

but if you have ever tried to stop eating added sugar and found it difficult, you are not alone. It is not all in your head.

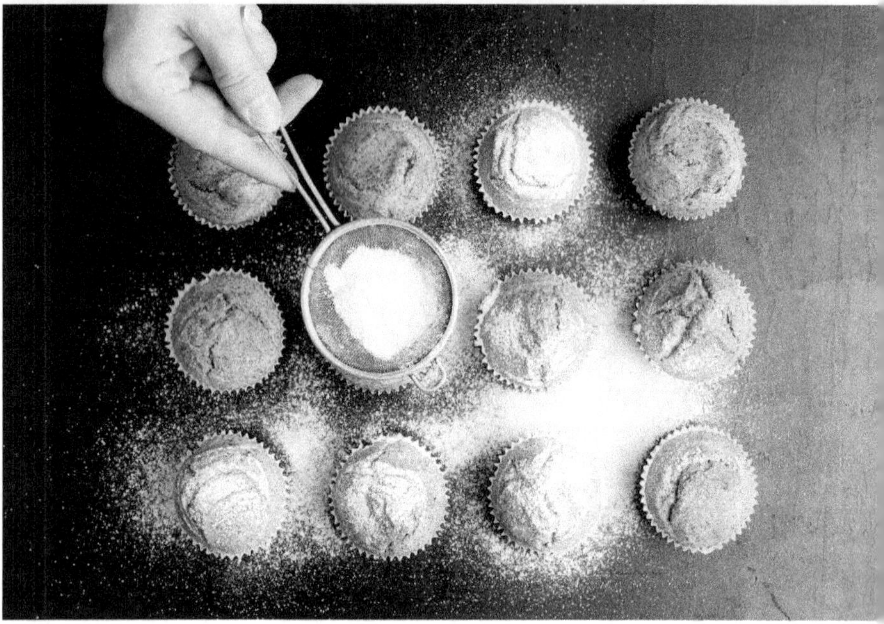

Unfortunately, the growing list of sugar substitutes and alternatives available nowadays does not solve the problem, as Dr. Hyman explains. Since many of today's sugar alternatives are 10-100 times sweeter than cane sugar, we quickly run the risk of overdoing it on even stronger stuff than good old cane sugar. We are wired to enjoy and seek out the taste of sweet thanks to evolutionary processes. Refined and added sugars oversaturate our taste buds without the fiber, vitamins, and minerals that nature normally packs into natural sources of sweetness such as fresh fruit or a subtly sweet yam or beet.

You may or may not find yourself in the following picture: many people sign up for a daylong roller coaster ride without even knowing it, and it has everything to do with sugar. The rollercoaster ride starts when they wake in the morning with low blood sugar. After a highly sweetened coffee drink loaded with hidden sugars, maybe paired with a sweetened morning pastry, blood sugar levels skyrocket. Not too long after, blood sugar levels drop as steeply and sharply as they skyrocketed, bringing with it a craving for instant energy, in other words, more sugar. And so the rollercoaster continues.

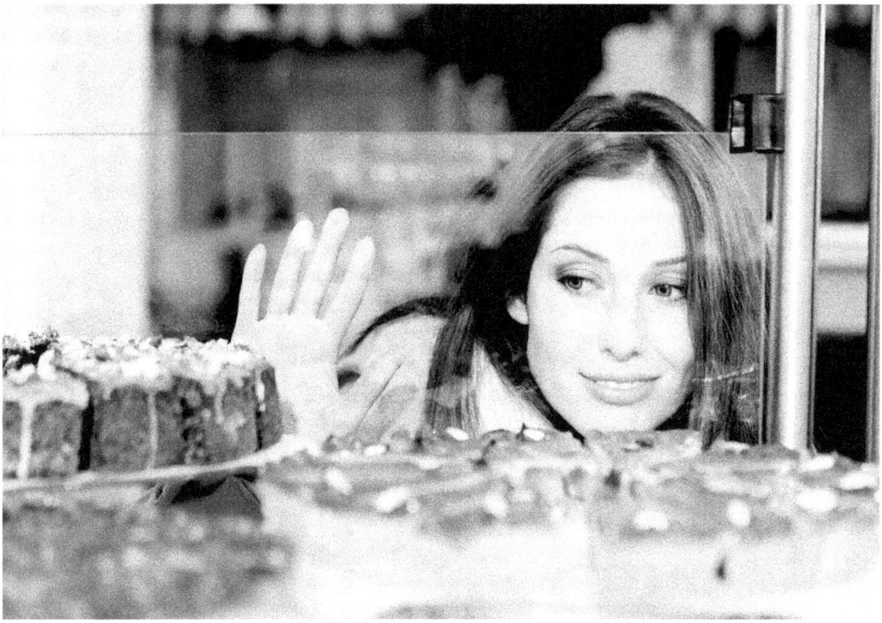

A spike in blood sugar triggers the release of insulin, the hormone that regulates blood sugar and stimulates hunger. Insulin also prompts the conversion and storage of sugar into fat. Sure, insulin transports much of the starches and sugars we consume into muscles for energy storage, but only when our stores are low and we are actively working hard like during intense exercise. For the majority of the day, the body doesn't know what to do with the continuous stream of sugars many of us eat throughout the day, so the body does what it does best – storing energy as fat to protect us from famine and hard times. Remember that insulin activates hunger signals, so it is no help that blood sugar spikes and consequent insulin spikes also lead to sudden

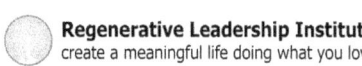

Regenerative Leadership Institute
create a meaningful life doing what you love

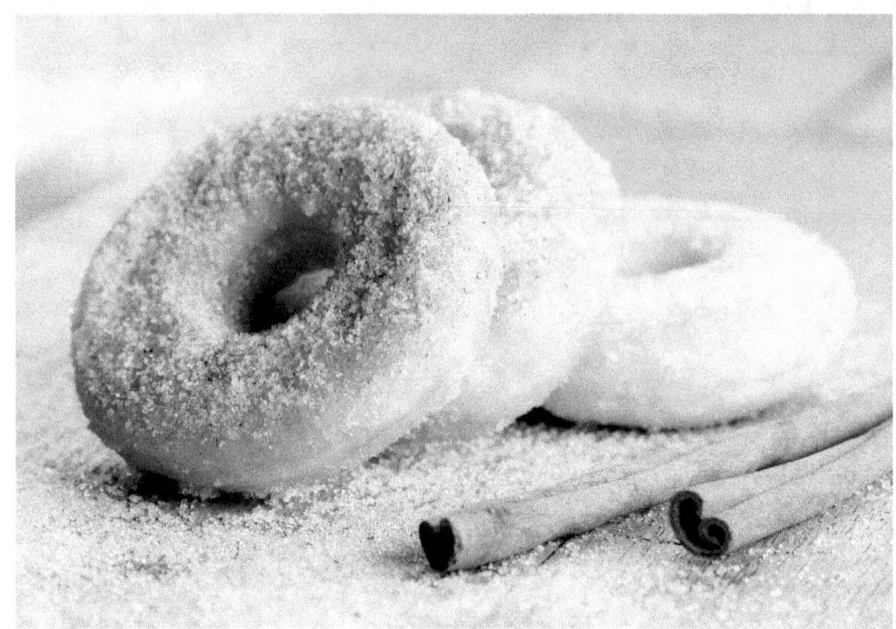

hunger pangs, at least some of which have more to do with imbalances in our diet and insulin response and less to do with genuine hunger and need for calories.

Sugar, and the simple carbohydrates that break down quickly to become sugars once we eat them, are not the whole story, but they are a big part of it. Glucose is what we call blood sugar. Whole grains, legumes, vegetables, soda, pastries – each of these has different kinds of carbohydrate, of which varying amounts break down and become blood glucose, or blood sugar, through the course of digestion. To be clear, our body requires a reliable supply of glucose, and steady blood sugar powers many critical systems in our body – the brain alone consumes up to one-fifth of our blood glucose, in fact! The determining factor is thus the effect of the overall package represented by a given food upon our blood sugar levels. The key nutrients, vitamins, minerals, and fiber that come along for the ride with that carbohydrate in a given food make all the difference.

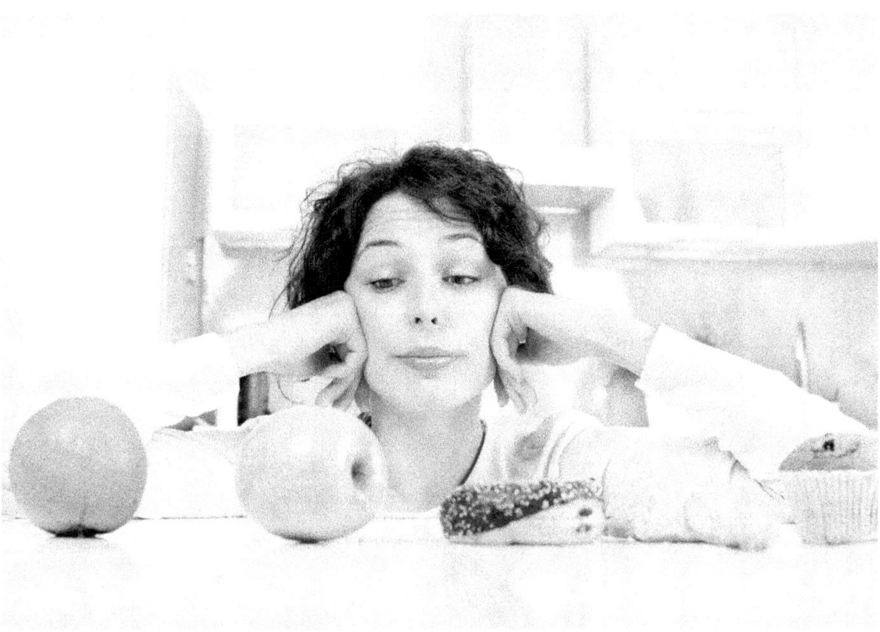

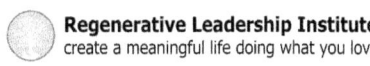

Why Diets & Deprivation Don't Work

News outlets routinely highlight the latest study suggesting that diets don't work. And anyone who has tried one likely has good insight into why that is.

Current research indicates that willpower is a finite resource. In studies where participants are left alone in a room with a cookie, following mentally demanding tasks, the individuals who tackled harder questions were less able to resist the cookie than the others who got the easy questions.

Translated to a dieting scenario, an individual's willpower to deprive themselves for the sake of their diet will decrease as the stressors and demands in his or her life increase. People often find it more challenging to muster the willpower to deprive themselves of foods they want or crave when they are already tired, low energy, stressed, anxious, depressed, or otherwise upset.

Regenerative Leadership Institute
create a meaningful life doing what you love

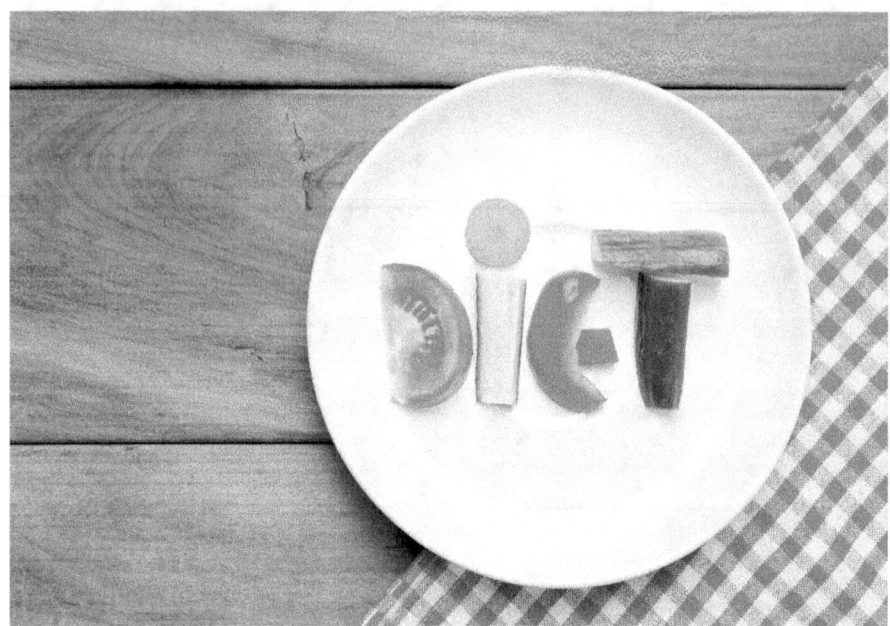

For many people, the word "diet" is synonymous with deprivation. A crash diet approach is popular, yet this short-term and sudden effort to lose weight or shift health indicators often involves sacrifices that the dieter never intends to maintain long-term. A dieter may even see desired results in the short term, but they rarely last for long because it is all too easy to return to pre-diet eating and lifestyle habits. This can leave someone even worse off than when they started the diet.

Deprivation and extreme calorie deficits can actually signal the body to respond as if it were responding to a famine. The body begins to operate differently in anticipation of the long stretch before food is available once again. Metabolism slows, and the body may even begin to break down muscle in its quest to survive the famine and to mobilize fuel. This is not the path to optimal health: don't forget that your ticker is comprised of muscle, too, and we all want our hearts to be as strong as possible!

Regenerative Leadership Institute
create a meaningful life doing what you love

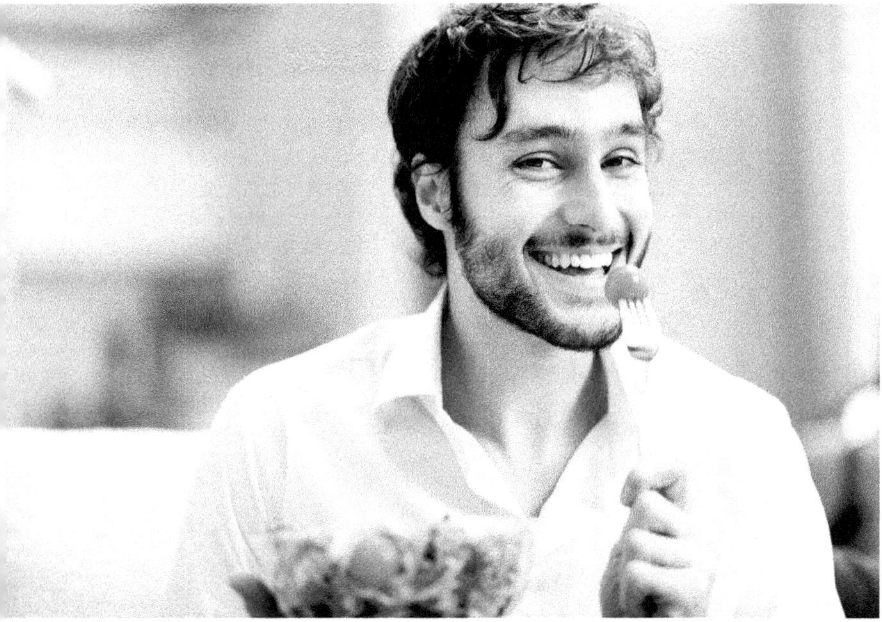

Crash diets and fad diets often rely on training individuals to cut out entire food groups with little explanation and minimal support to find realistic and healthy substitutes. It is also quite routine for the average crash dieter to develop guilt and shame, a sense of right and wrong, when it comes to their deprivation strategies. This is really harmful both physically and psychologically. If you have had any history with crash and fad diets, you have felt their effects firsthand, and you know the damage an omnipresent sense of deprivation can do.

Instead, our approach here is refreshingly different:
- learn the power of whole nutrient-dense foods for yourself
- appreciate the benefits of these foods for your short and long-term health
- understand the risks associated with the Standard American Diet by contrast
- make gradual changes to your eating habits to avoid overwhelm and see for yourself how much better you feel

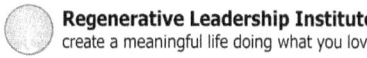

Regenerative Leadership Institute
create a meaningful life doing what you love

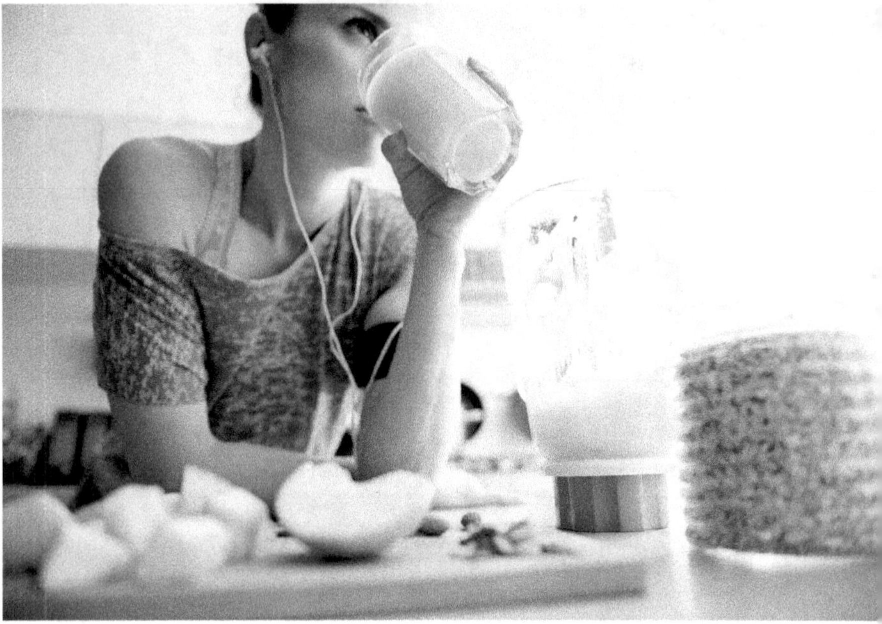

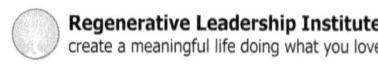

- add in more of the good stuff, and skip the worrying about do and don't lists or judging yourself for falling off track at a meal

Think *"Fall down seven times, get up eight"* (Japanese proverb). Not *"No pain, no gain."* Got it?

The Way Forward

"He that takes medicine and neglects diet, wastes the skills of the physician."
Chinese proverb

Maybe that bit about falling down seven times still gets you down and sounds a little bleak. **But wait, there is hope!**

Regenerative Leadership Institute
create a meaningful life doing what you love

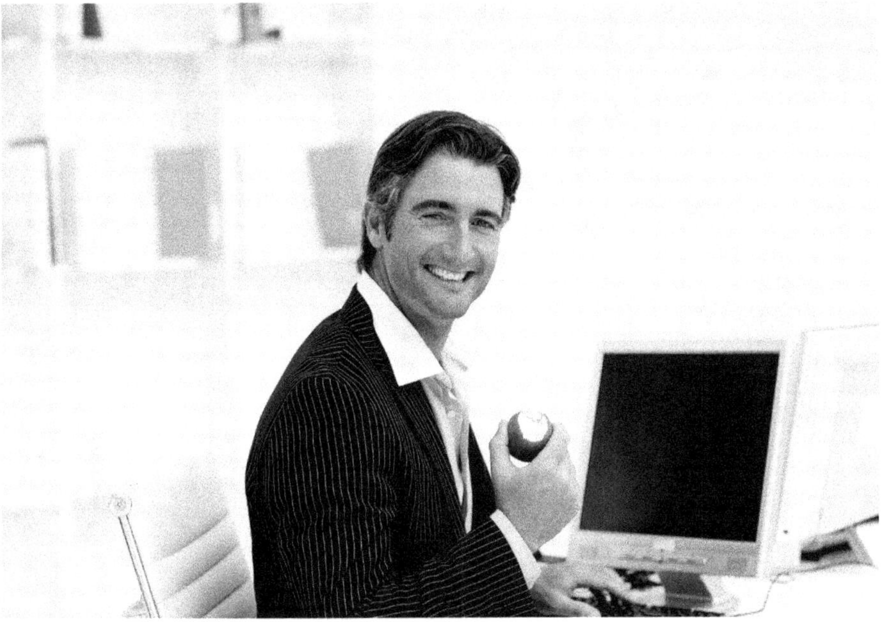

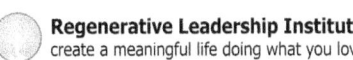

Remember that part about lifestyle and diet as the most influential determinants of your health? Well, believe it or not, this is actually really *great* news. Because who has control over those? You do!

You have the power, and we'll show you the way, to make changes that lead you toward more vitality than you thought possible, more energy than you had yesterday, and a leaner, healthier you.

You may have spent the first many years of your life to establish your habits, so it usually doesn't last if you try to change *everything* all at once. However, small steps really do add up, and they stick. ***Our habits are learned and acquired, not permanent and hopelessly unalterable. With consistent effort and a little patience on your part, and guidance on the what, why, and how from us, you can and will transform the habits you wish to change and adopt healthier ones along the way.***

Regenerative Leadership Institute
create a meaningful life doing what you love

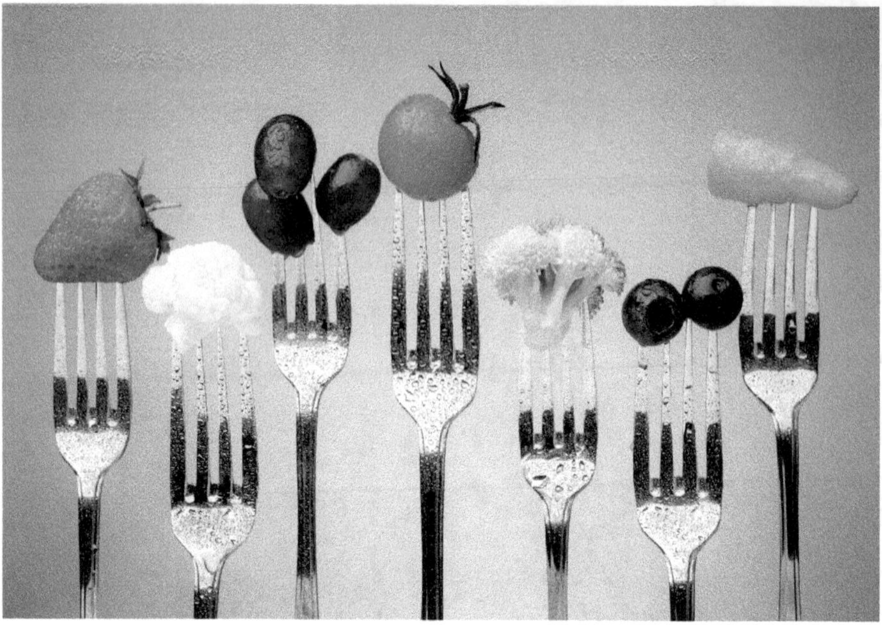

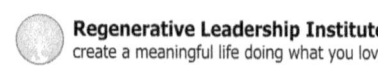

Even better, you will soon see that healthy eating is its own reward. Sure, it will feel new and unfamiliar at first, just like with any other change you make to your habits and routines. A huge advantage to the whole food, plant-based approach, though, is that its effects on energy, blood sugar, sleep, digestion, and more take hold rather quickly. Don't bother taking our word for it when it comes to feeling better when you eat this way. You'll see for yourself in a matter of weeks how nourishing it feels to choose real, whole foods in their most natural state. This way of eating creates a positive feedback loop on itself. This leads to further momentum and motivation to stick with this approach and adopt it as a lifestyle for the long term!

Lifestyle and diet modifications are as effective as medications, if not more potent, for many chronic diseases. The American College of Lifestyle Medicine has been around since 2004, and this specialty association for clinicians advocates the creation of a new specialty board certification in Lifestyle Medicine. That is how powerful and renowned lifestyle interventions can be, and this notion is at the heart of the approach of this book and our 8-week course.

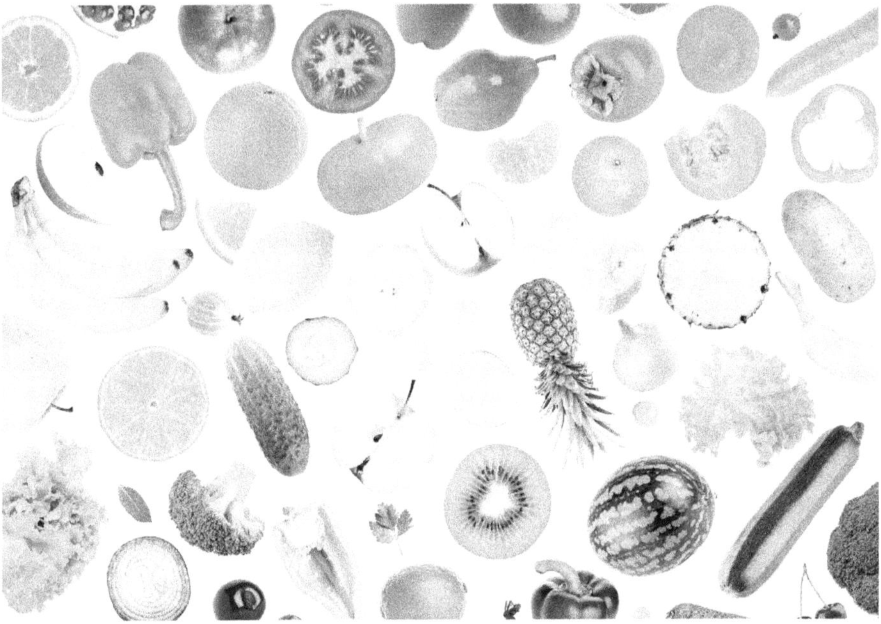

Lasting lifestyle and dietary change looks like gradual and consistent change that you can keep up with for the rest of your life, no crash diet or fad diet here. Make intentional, thoughtful changes in a way that truly works for you, and they are far more likely to last.

Low-Glycemic is Key

More good news! Yes, thank goodness.

Our whole food, plant-based approach to eating is inherently *low-glycemic*, and that is really, really good news.

First, some definitions: you may have heard terms like *glycemic index* and *glycemic* load before, and you may have become frustrated by

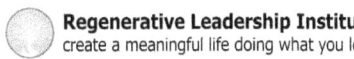

Regenerative Leadership Institute
create a meaningful life doing what you love

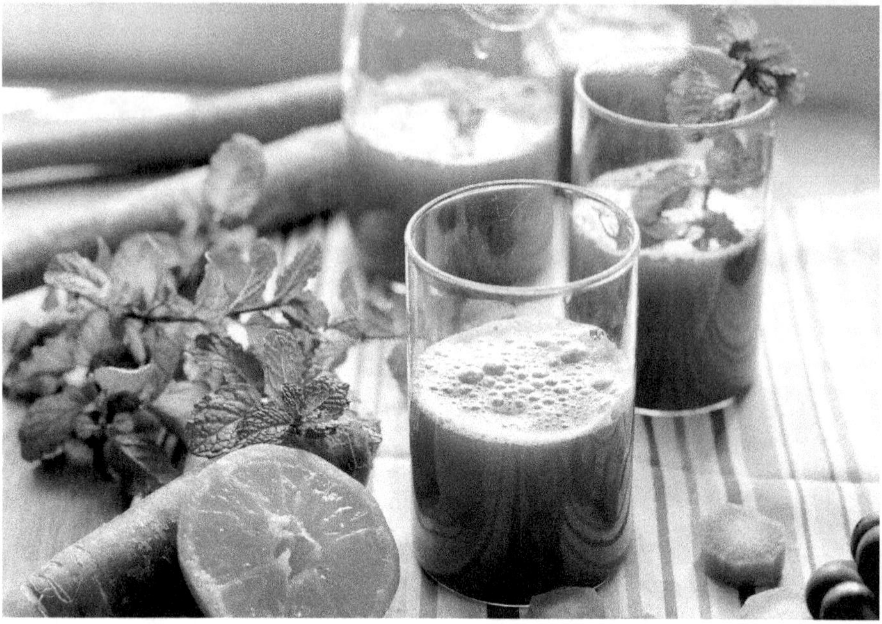

confusing definitions and conflicting information. Simply put, these terms are concerned with how food affects blood sugar. Glycemic index (GI) describes the effect of a given food's carbohydrates on blood sugar, since carbohydrates actually come in many forms, some better for us than others. A more recently developed measure, glycemic load (GL) evaluates both the particular carbohydrates in a given food along with the amount of those carbohydrates present in a typical serving size of that given food. This additional data point results in more realistic and accurate information, so the glycemic load of a given food provides a more complete picture of its impact on our blood sugar.

Now, apply the concept of glycemic load to whole food, plant-based eating. Generally speaking, the less processed and refined a food, the longer your body takes to digest it. It may sound strange, but you actually want your body to expend some energy to digest and break down your food. The longer it takes for the body to digest your lunch, the slower the glucose from the meal will hit the bloodstream, and

Regenerative Leadership Institute
create a meaningful life doing what you love

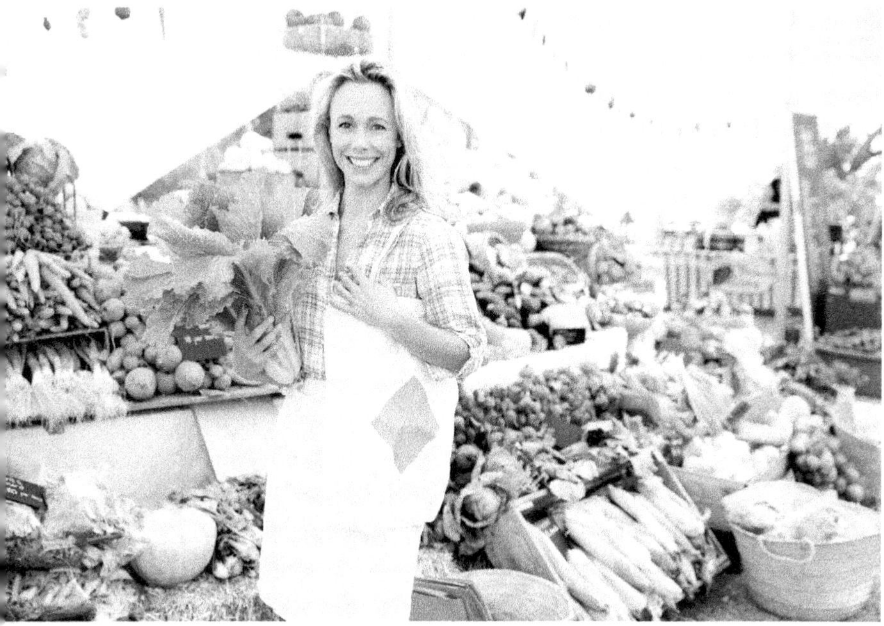

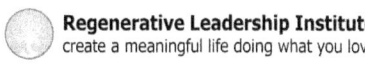

this results in a steady stream of energy. This is a far cry from the sharp spike and steep decline in blood sugar that occurs after we eat something that has quickly and easily absorbable sugars. Extensively processed and refined food may be appropriately described as pre-digested food. As gross as this may sound, there is some truth in this: the more we grind up, preserve, press into oils, dehydrate, fry and roast, separate and isolate, and add preservatives and stabilizers, the less time and effort required by our body to break apart the food and absorb the necessary nutrients. It is preferable that our bodies spend time and energy to sort through and benefit from the fiber, water, vitamins, and minerals present in whole, intact foods. By contrast, processed and packaged foods have usually been stripped of the fiber, water, vitamins and/or minerals in order to extend shelf life and supersize flavor to encourage larger portions and cravings.

To disembark from the sugar rollercoaster for good, to regain control over your blood sugar, energy level, and mood, emphasize whole

Regenerative Leadership Institute
create a meaningful life doing what you love

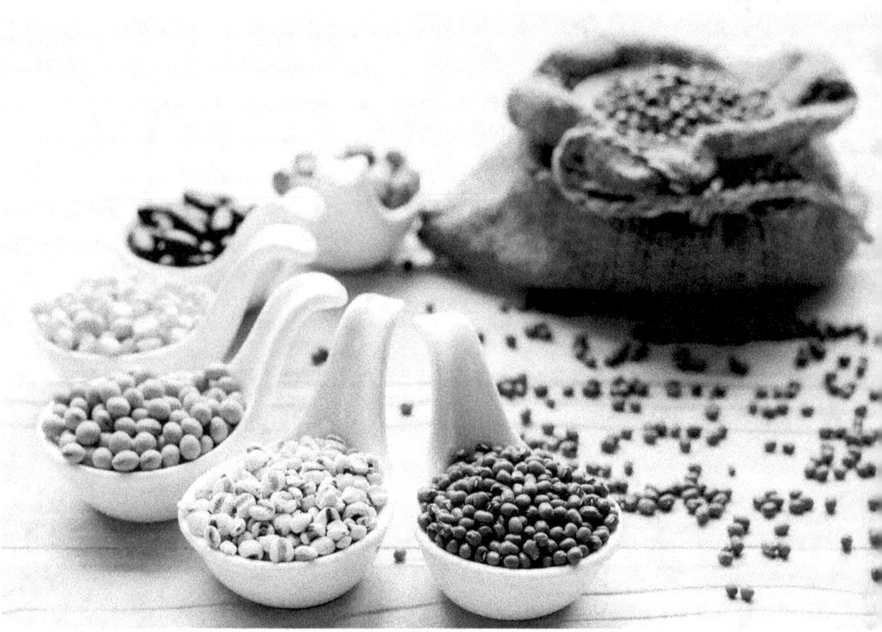

foods in their most original and intact form as often as you can. Fruits and vegetables, legumes, nuts, seeds, whole grains – load up on these whole, plant-based foods whether you are cooking at home or making healthful selections when dining out. This is low-glycemic eating made easy, no calorie counting or serving size calculators required.

Evidence abounds for the positive impact of low-glycemic eating on our long-term health. This simple eating plan has been shown to:
- decrease HbA1c levels in people with diabetes
- improve blood sugar management and decrease insulin resistance in people at high risk of diabetes
- reduce risk of various inflammatory processes such as deteriorating endothelial function characteristic of heart disease
- lower high blood pressure (low-glycemic eating is already a component of the highly regarded and established DASH, or, Dietary Approaches to Stop Hypertension, promoted by the National Institutes of Health
- contribute to healthy and sustainable weight loss that lasts

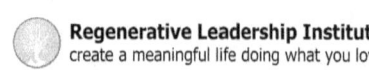
Regenerative Leadership Institute
create a meaningful life doing what you love

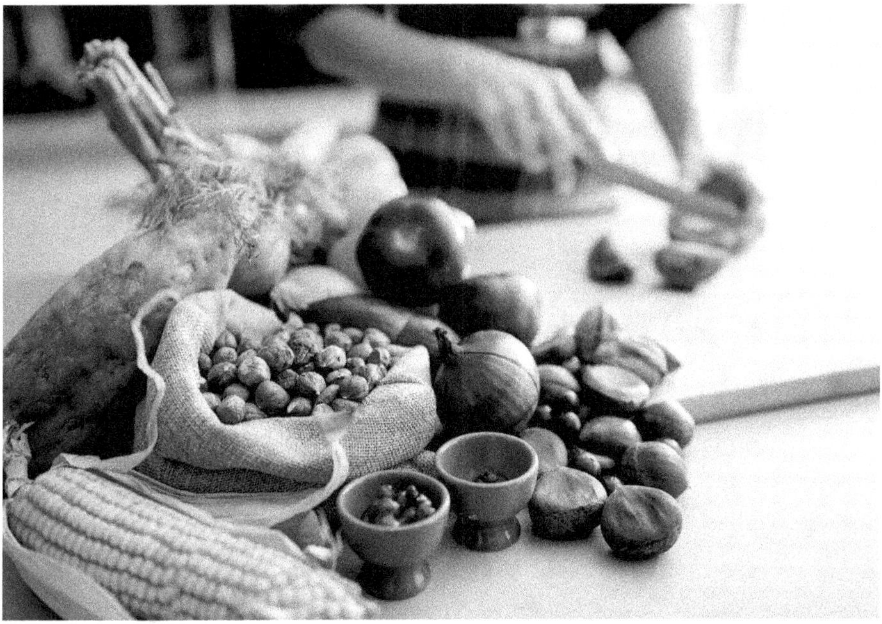

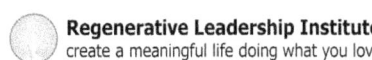

- reduce the liver's buildup of fat associated with non-alcoholic fatty liver disease.

As if that weren't enough, many people come to prefer low-glycemic meals and snacks for their satiety factor – people feel full for longer when eating this way. In case you want to lose extra weight, or boost your energy, or cut back on mindless snacking, low-glycemic eating is the strategy you have been searching for. Read on for much, much more about this approach, and learn how to implement this lifestyle step-by-step in our 8-week course!

Small Steps

"It is better to take many small steps in the right direction than to make a great leap forward only to stumble backward."

Chinese proverb

Regenerative Leadership Institute
create a meaningful life doing what you love

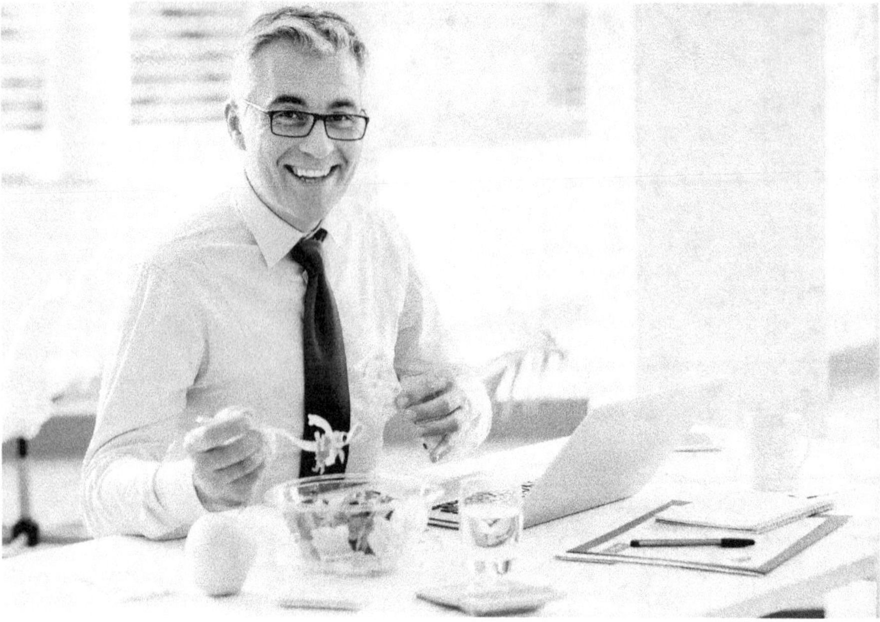

Small steps add up. That fact is the foundation of our approach during the *60 Days To A Healthier Life* 8-week course. We invite you to focus on just a few small changes at a time, rather than expect yourself to wake up tomorrow to brand new habits in the areas you want to change.

In fact, this approach suits any ambitious goal. How do you hand wash a sink full of dishes? One dish at a time. How do you wash a sink full of dishes if you have a dishwasher? Still, one step at a time: load it until full, add the detergent, hit "start," wait for it to finish, then unload one or two plates at a time.

As you succeed at each small step, you create actual change, and you build confidence at the same time. The steps you start with in Week One are nearly second nature by Week Five.

In fact, in our 8-week course, the first several steps and recommendations are designed to be easier and more accessible. These first steps serve

Regenerative Leadership Institute
create a meaningful life doing what you love

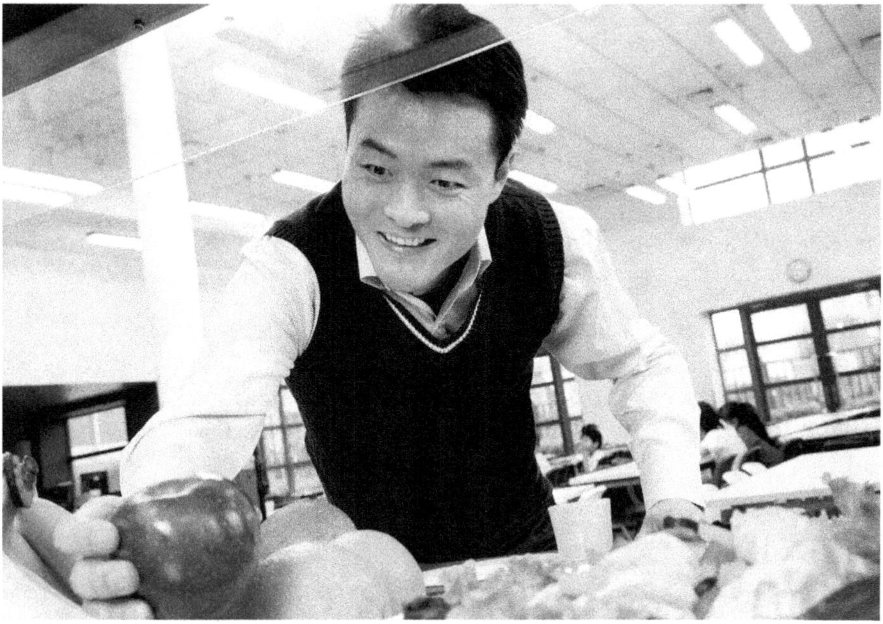

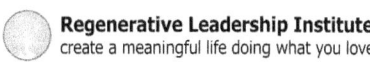

as a warm-up to the rest of the course and to the larger task of making this stick as a lifestyle. But, first things first, take small and consistent steps to make changes to your eating habits and other behaviors that will last you a lifetime.

Even small steps create immediate change. Depending on your situation, you may even see significant impact from just one change. As you get off that sugar roller coaster, if you're on it now, the first few days might be rough. But before the week is out, you may notice fewer mood swings, more consistency and control over your energy levels, fewer cravings, and other changes!

Specifically on weight loss, despite what we all see on television shows like The Biggest Loser, lasting weight loss is typically a gradual process. Every inch closer to your healthiest weight improves many other aspects of your health along the way: blood pressure, cholesterol, blood sugar management, triglycerides, chronic conditions, energy, stress, sleep, and more!

Regenerative Leadership Institute
create a meaningful life doing what you love

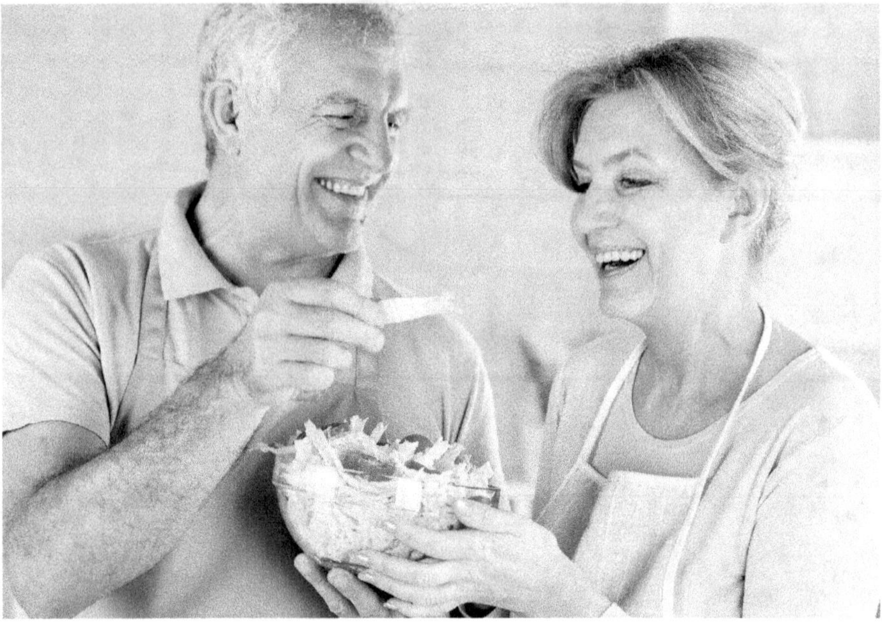

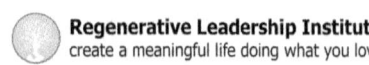

It is less like an instant on/off switch and more like a gradual slide along a spectrum toward optimal health.

The Answer

"By treating the root causes of diseases with plants not pills, we can also avoid the adverse side effects of prescription drugs that kill more than 100,000 Americans every year, making them a leading cause of death."

Michael Greger, MD, family physician, author, and internationally known speaker on food safety, nutrition, and public health issues

We know you are committed to your own health and happiness: you wouldn't be reading this is if you weren't. This book and our 8-week course equips you to take charge of your health, achieve your desired results, and pursue your own health and happiness as comfortably as possible!

Regenerative Leadership Institute
create a meaningful life doing what you love

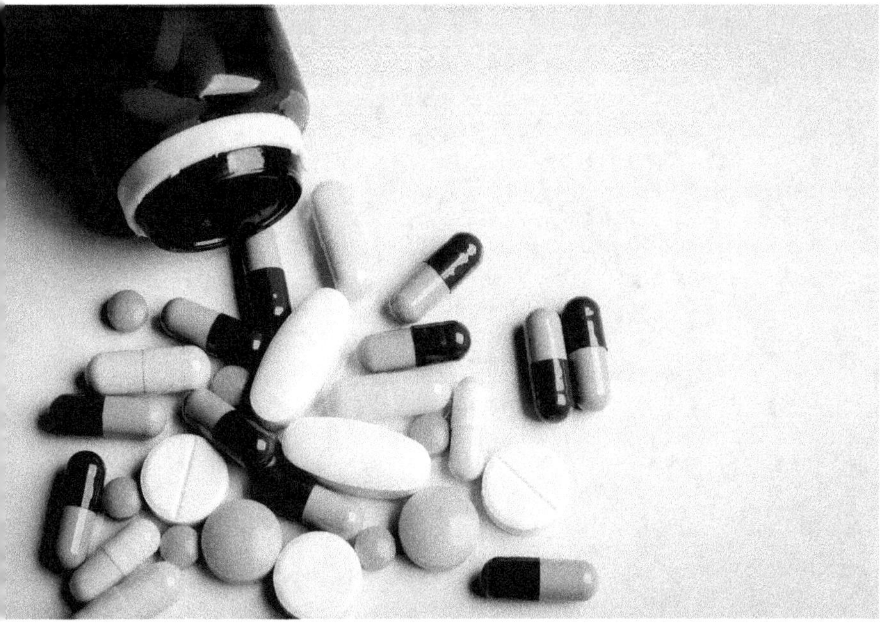

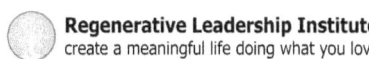

Here's your special invitation: **welcome to the whole food, plant-based way of eating and living!** Clinical research has already shown that this is an effective path for many people to lose weight, improve health numbers, feel better, and outmaneuver many of the "diet and lifestyle diseases" we mentioned earlier.

Outsmart and lower your risk for developing lifestyle diseases, better manage and even possibly reverse a chronic condition – how can this be possible? We certainly don't toss around these phrases lightly. It sounds too good to be true: a whole food, plant-based eating plan has a fast-growing body of evidence to support these claims. The best part is that it is relatively easy, inexpensive, and far less invasive compared to other standard recommendations such as strong prescription medications for life, or surgeries and other medical procedures.

Think of it this way: isn't it worth a try? You won't find another approach with such compelling evidence and claims of effectiveness against a

Regenerative Leadership Institute
create a meaningful life doing what you love

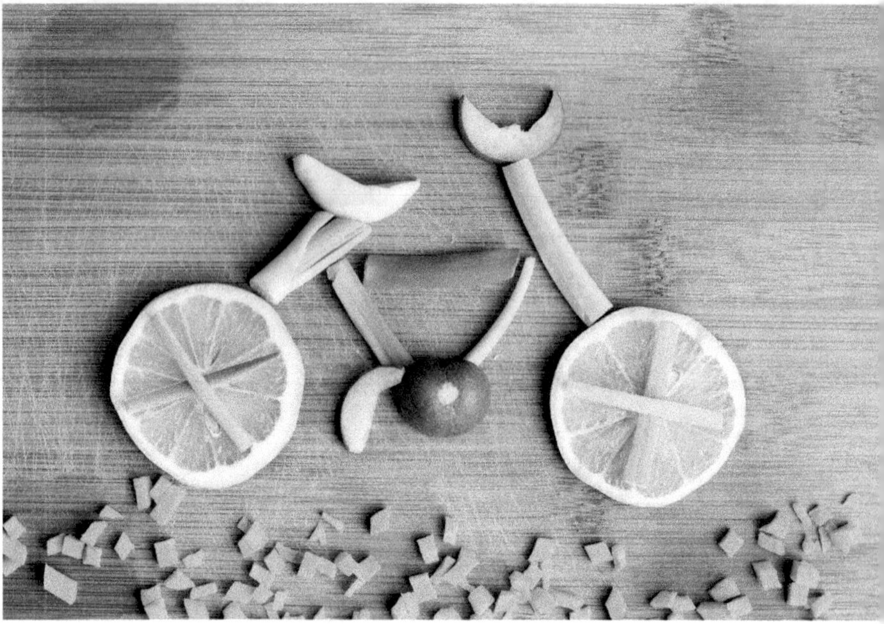

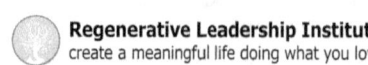

variety of maladies and chronic conditions that is easier on the wallet or your body, for that matter. A colorful spectrum of whole fruits and vegetables, foods rich with vitamins, minerals, and enzymes – these are the foods you treat yourself to when you eat with us!

What It Looks Like

This approach will be less of a change than you expect. Take a moment – yes, right now! – to look at your refrigerator, freezer, and pantry shelves, something you have done countless times before. But, this time, you are looking for plant-based foods! You certainly already have many, many plant-based foods on your plate and in your grocery cart, whether you realize it or not.

This list is most certainly not exhaustive, but it's a start!
- **Fruits,** fresh or frozen (apples, oranges, bananas, pineapple, berries, grapefruit, melon, peaches, pears, plums, coconut, avocadoes and

Regenerative Leadership Institute
create a meaningful life doing what you love

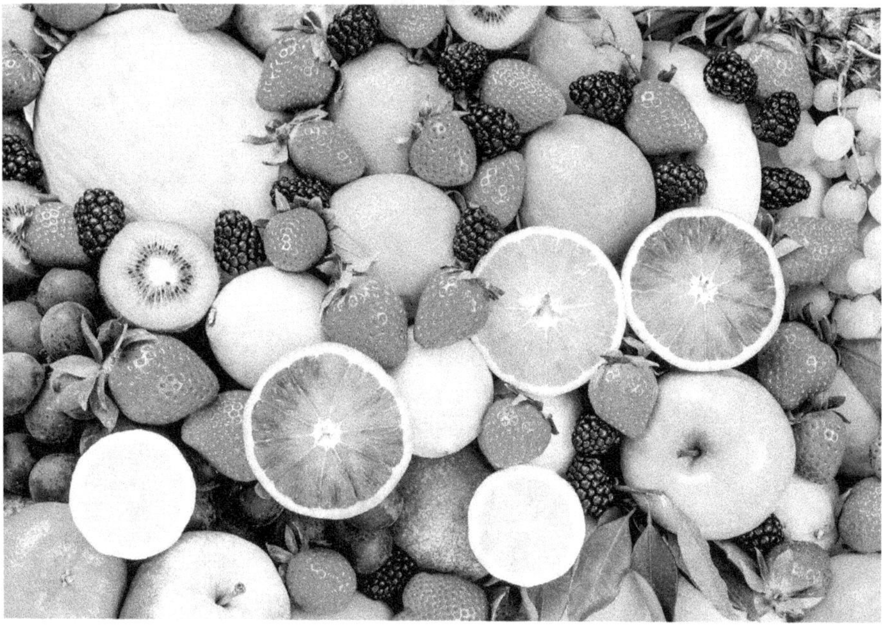

![fruits and berries]

olives [yes, those last three are technically fruit!]...)
- **Vegetables,** fresh or frozen (carrot, bell pepper, broccoli, corn, peas, jicama, sweet potatoes, artichoke, bok choy, tomatoes, spinach, iceberg lettuce, pumpkin, kale, cauliflower, onion, garlic, cabbage, mushrooms, sea vegetables...)
- **Nuts** (almonds, cashews, walnuts, pistachios, peanuts, nut butters...)
- **Seeds** (sunflower, sesame, pumpkin, quinoa, amaranth, hemp, chia, flax...)
- **Grains and cereals,** in their whole and intact form (oats, rice, millet, barley...)
- **Spices, herbs and seasonings,** fresh or dried (parsley, rosemary, mint, basil, cilantro, salt, pepper, cumin, chili pepper...)
- **Legumes** (black beans, pinto beans, garbanzos, lentils, black-eyed peas, split peas...)

Plus, when you dine out with friends and family, it is easy to find healthful plant-based items that fit the bill. Just a few examples to inspire your

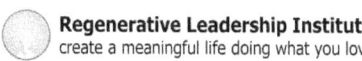

Regenerative Leadership Institute
create a meaningful life doing what you love

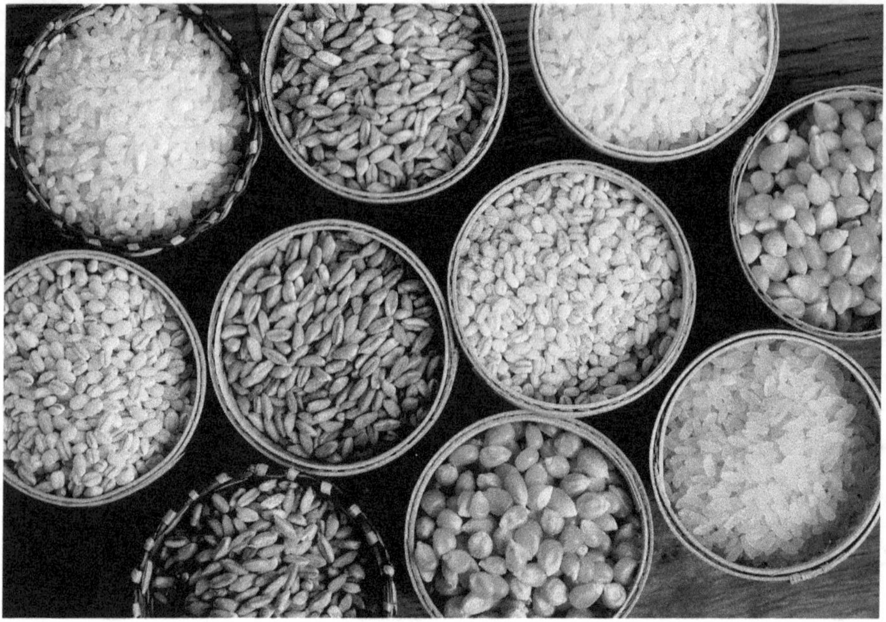

creative thinking when you go out to your next meal. Again, this is not an exhaustive list, there are many more great examples of plant-based meals when you look for them!

- Burritos, tacos, or bowls loaded with beans and rice, vegetables, salsa and guacamole at Mexican or other Latin American restaurants
- Coconut milk-based curries, dishes featuring eggplant or beans or potatoes in non-dairy sauces at Indian restaurants
- A huge plate of steamed vegetables or a stir-fry rice dish loaded with vegetables, or fresh spring rolls or veggie dumplings
- Hummus, babaganoush, lentil dishes, and falafels at Mediterranean and Middle Eastern restaurants
- Sandwich bursting with veggies and other fillings: lettuce, tomato, artichoke, olive, cucumber, sprouts, hummus, sundried tomato, avocado, and mustard at a sandwich place
- Even pizza joints will often cater to your requests to double the vegetable toppings and sauce but hold the cheese

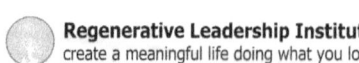

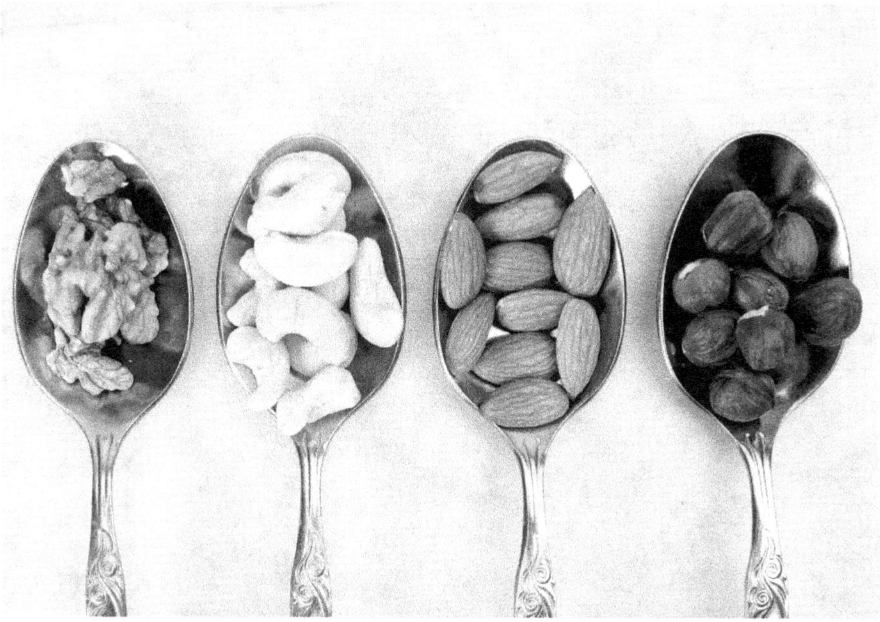

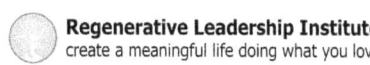

- Steamed, roasted, or grilled vegetables with marinara sauce or fresh tomatoes and a little olive oil, with a double side salad at an Italian restaurant.

Among the advantages of a whole food, plant-based eating plan is the sheer variety of colors, flavors, and textures you will find on your plate. Whole food, plant-based cuisine is arguably more creative and unorthodox, often intentionally designed to hit as many of our five tastes – sweet, salty, sour, bitter, and umami – as possible. If you seek out restaurants that cater to this cuisine, you will find that these chefs are incredibly creative with their dishes and pairings because they know that many of their diners could be in tastebud transition and may still seek the flavors associated with familiar animal-based foods.

It is worth noting that many of the flavors we associate with animal-based foods and many popular items on the S.A.D. menu are not unique to those foods. Are you a cheese connoisseur, for instance? If you are, you probably appreciate the salty and complex cultured flavor of cheeses. Did you know you can recreate those flavors by allowing plant-based cheeses to culture in a similar fashion? A simple recipe of cashews, water, culture, and desired salt and spices left to ferment for a period of hours or days yields a remarkably complex flavor. This is only one example, as plant-based cheeses can be made from a variety of starting ingredients. All kinds of techniques exist to achieve the consistencies associated with dairy cheeses from whipped cream cheese-like texture to dense, hard, cheesewheel-like texture.

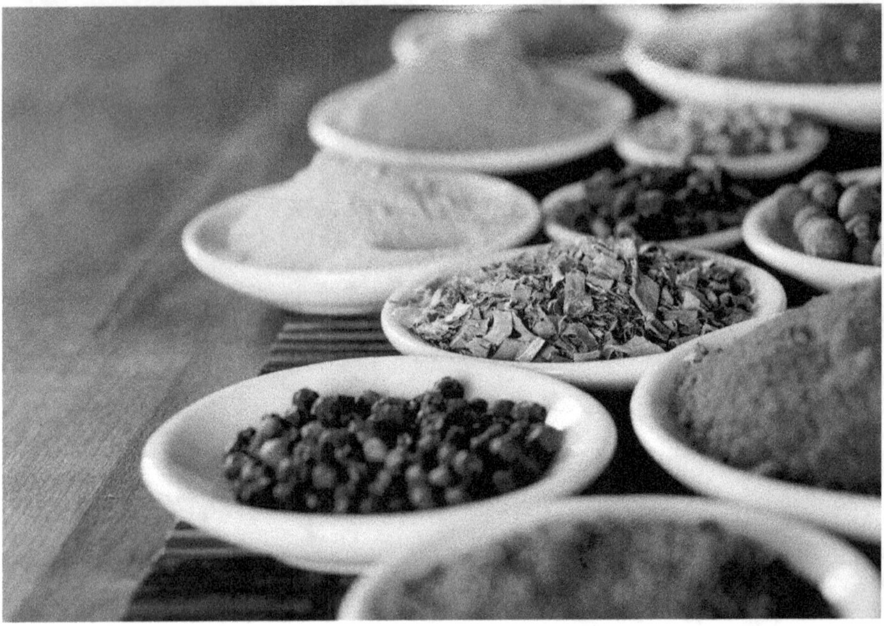

It is also worth noting that our tastebuds in fact change and respond to what we eat. If you eat mostly packaged and processed foods right now, you will notice that the salt and sugar are missing from a plate of steamed vegetables or an unseasoned stir fry, for instance. An example: if table sugar and ice cream are the sweetest foods in Rob's current diet, his tastebuds adapt to read those as sweet

Regenerative Leadership Institute
create a meaningful life doing what you love

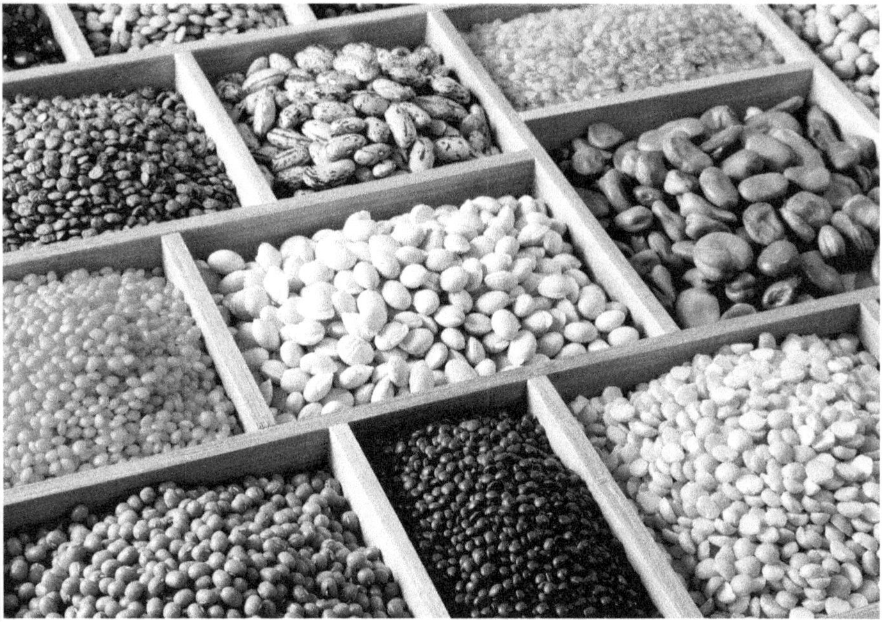

and read everything else as less sweet. The extremes of our diet, however healthy or unhealthy they are, become the benchmark for our tastebuds to recognize sweet. Now, let's say Rob signs up for our 8-week course and continues to remove added sugars from his diet and replace them with whole food sources of sweetness such as fresh fruit, and sometimes frozen and dried fruit. Within a week or two, an overripe banana or a plump raisin will feel like a special sweet treat to his tastebuds because he has established a new benchmark for sweet. If he returns to sprinkling table sugar over his morning cereal or a scoop of ice cream, he may even find them overly sweet and not nearly as appealing as they used to be.

When we take a leap of faith and explore a whole food, plant-based way of eating, we are often pleasantly surprised that our tastebuds adapt and even inspire us to appreciate whole foods in a new light. Sure, bananas and raisins and many fruits will taste sweeter than ever to you, but other foods will surprise you and taste sweeter than you

Regenerative Leadership Institute
create a meaningful life doing what you love

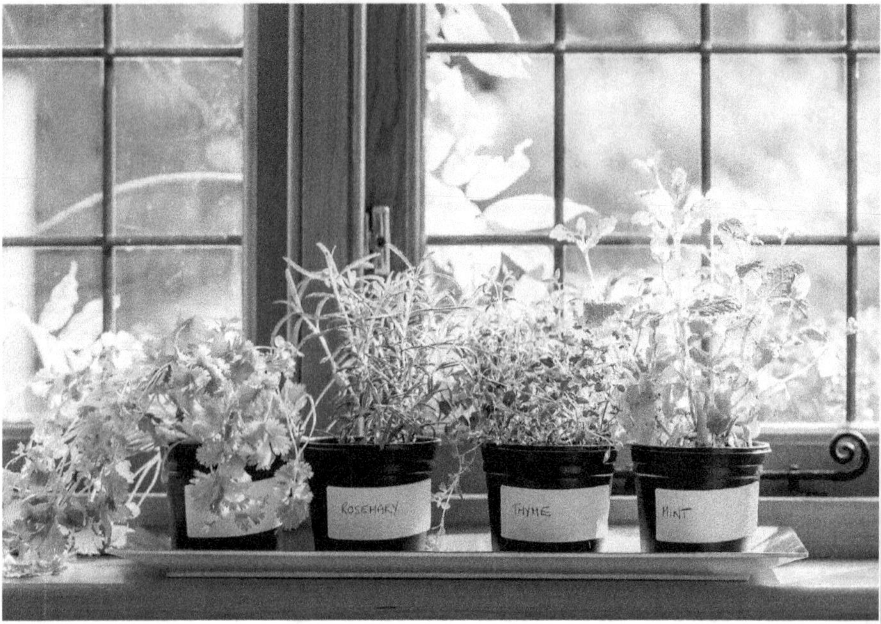

ever remembered them, too. After making changes like this, many people are surprised to detect the sweet taste of carrots, corn, beets, sweet potatoes, even cooked greens!

Many more natural and delicious alternatives exist to dress a plate of vegetables for less or no sodium and no added sugars, but you still might detect a contrast from the soy sauce marinade packet that accompanies the average package of frozen stir fry vegetables from the grocery store, or the teriyaki marinated rice bowl at your favorite restaurant.

However, in a matter of a week or two, your tastebuds actually shift according to what is on your plate.

Day In The Life: A Sample Day's Meal Plan

Better yet, this day-long meal plan shows you how easy and tasty it can be to throw together meals centered around whole plant-based foods.

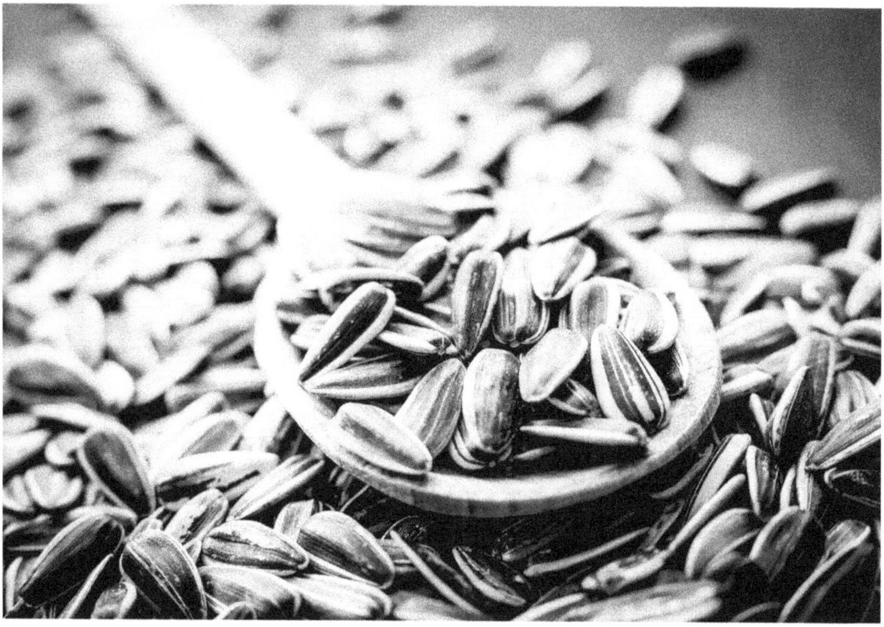

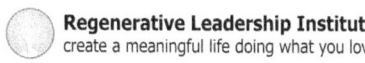

BREAKFAST IDEAS – Don't forget to grab 2 or more pieces of fresh fruit on your way out the door for easy snacks throughout the day!

• *Chia seed pudding* - chia seeds soaked in water or plant-based milk (ratio of 6 parts liquid to 1 part chia) in the refrigerator overnight. Add generous amounts of cinnamon, vanilla extract, and/or any other spices you like. Add your favorite chopped nuts like walnuts, freshly sliced fruit like banana, and other desired toppings just before serving.

• *Steaming bowl of oatmeal* simply cooked in water and topped with chopped fresh fruit like bananas, berries, apples, or your favorite fruit. Add a tablespoon of ground flax seeds, whole chia seeds, or hulled hemp seeds for more protein and healthy fats. Sprinkle cinnamon, cloves, or other desired spices. Add your favorite chopped nuts for more healthy fats and keep you feeling full until lunch. You can actually make a porridge out of any leftover grain you like – leftover cooked rice, quinoa, millet, etc – by simmering the cooked grain for

Regenerative Leadership Institute
create a meaningful life doing what you love

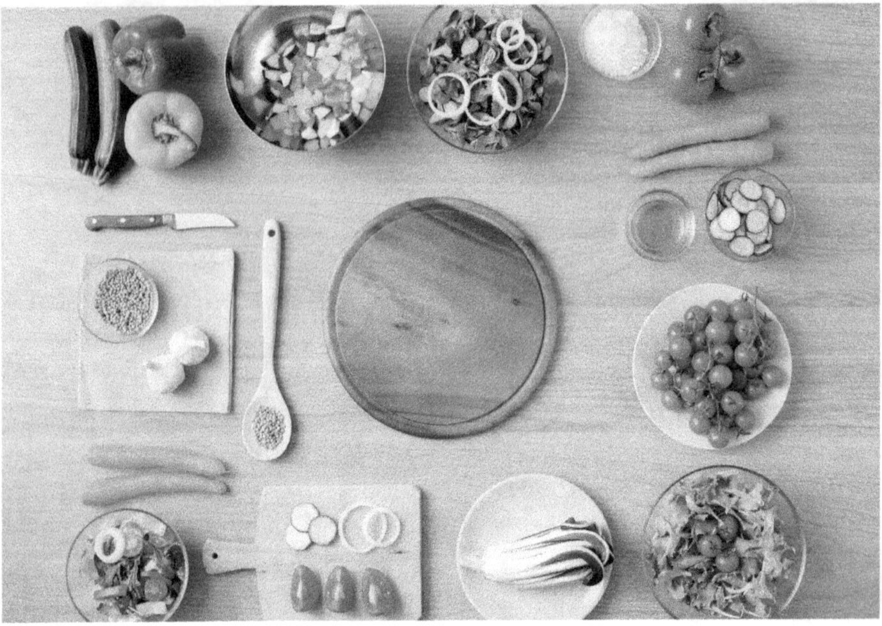

![Salad ingredients arranged around an empty wooden plate]

a few minutes and adding the above toppings. You can even make a raw muesli or parfait by mixing and matching the above ingredients – fruit, seeds, nuts, spices, even add shredded unsweetened coconut!

LUNCH – Load up your plate! We are often accustomed to side salads, but when salad is the main attraction, you can really load up your plate and have a generous serving because this likely totals far fewer calories than your standard lunch fare.

· *Big, huge salad with all the fixings* - think salad bar-style! Start with your base of greens and mix it up from week to week to try new tastes and find your favorite: iceberg, romaine, spinach, arugula, kale... Generous serving of beans (or mix and match +1 kind), finely diced veggies like tomatoes, cucumber, carrots, green peas, red onion, corn, jicama, mushrooms, bell pepper, and other favorite veggies. Don't forget to add something that provides healthy fats for more nutrition and satiety: think avocado, olives, and/or nuts. A sprinkle of chopped fresh or dried fruit also makes a great

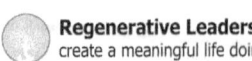

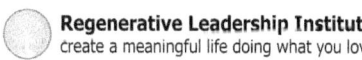

and satisfying addition. Dress with lemon juice + gluten-free tamari, or apple cider vinegar/balsamic vinegar + dash of olive oil, e.g.

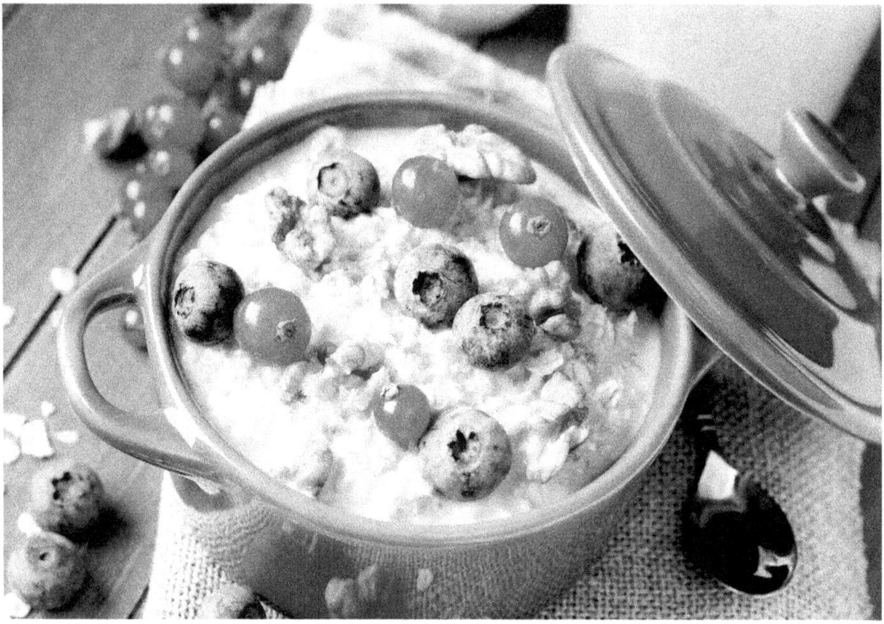

DINNER – Load up your plate, again!

· *Hearty, tabouleh-style quinoa plate* – dressed with a tahini/lemon juice/cumin/minced garlic dressing and topped with sliced radishes, chickpeas, minced parsley, diced celery and carrots, olives or capers. Garnish with a few sliced almonds and a sprinkling of fresh or dried fruit on top - try currants, raisins, or dried apricots on top. Add a steamed sweet potato for a filling meal. Add other seasonal vegetables as desired. Make a big batch so that you can take leftovers for lunch tomorrow!

DESSERT

· *Stuffed dates* – add your favorite nut or teaspoon of nut butter inside the date. If you go with nut butter, look for unsalted, raw, and no added sugars or oils because it's better for you that way!). If using nuts instead, pecans, walnuts, cashews, and almonds are great for this! Sprinkle unsweetened shredded coconut on top if you like. Sprinkle cinnamon on top, even a tiny pinch of sea salt, for a caramel-like salty+sweet taste!

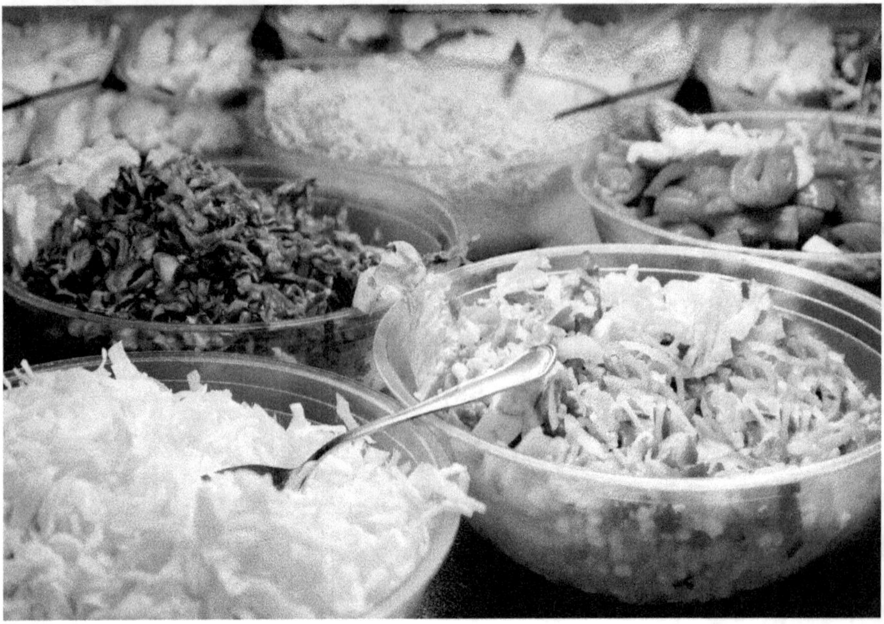

SNACK on fresh and dried fruit and nuts, or raw veggies and dip like hummus or guacamole. If you have a minute, make a smoothie with fresh or frozen fruit, a spoonful of nut butter or nuts, a big handful of tender greens like spinach or baby kale or even romaine lettuce, and a cup of cold water or juice!

Guiding Principles

There is absolutely no reason this has to be a difficult transition. Some of the leading advocates of plant-based lifestyles were themselves

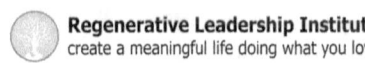
Regenerative Leadership Institute
create a meaningful life doing what you love

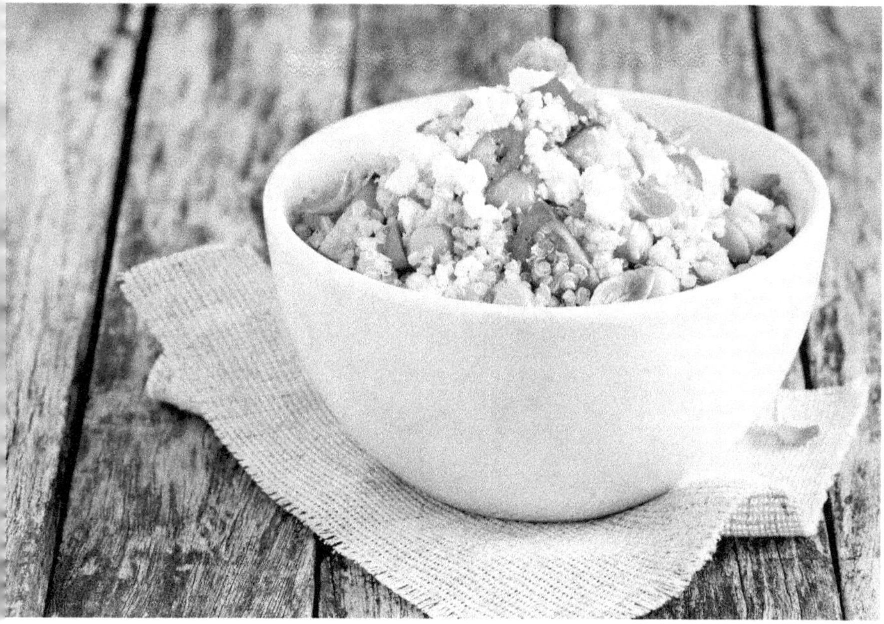

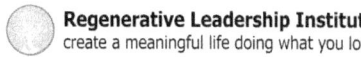

raised on dairy farms and cattle ranches! If they can make this change, so can you. What does "whole food, plant-based way of eating" actually mean? The short answer: choose foods that come from plants in their least processed, most original and intact form.

These five principles will guide you on your journey to a healthier life and weight:
1. From processed foods to whole foods
2. From animal foods to plant foods
3. From quantity to quality
4. From mindless eating to mindful eating
5. It's about what you CAN eat, not what you can't

Let's dig into each of these, so you understand what we mean beyond the sound bite.

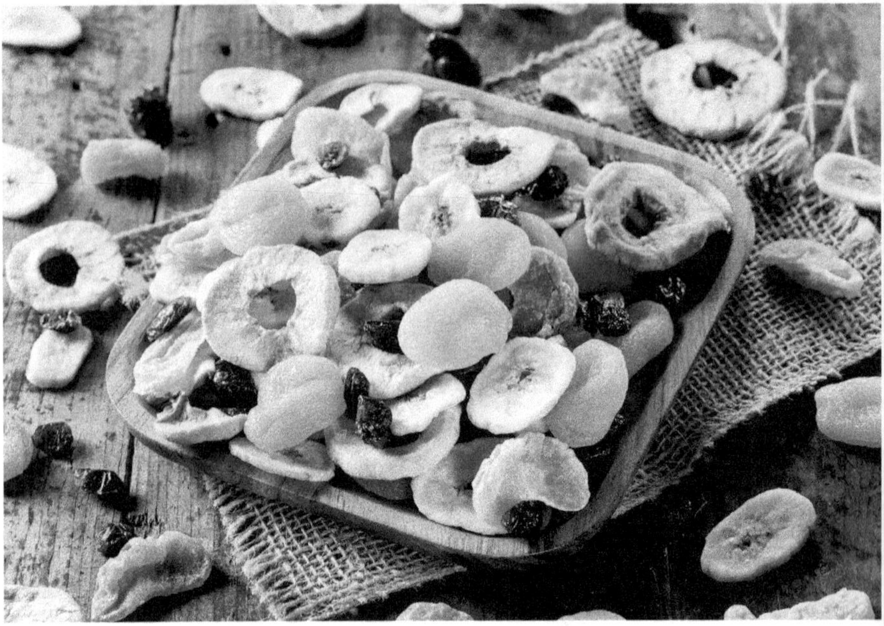

From Processed Foods to Whole Foods

"I've long been a dedicated student of food labels, and it's really quite shocking that some breakfast cereals are much saltier than salty snacks. And some pasta sauces have much more added sugar than ice cream toppings."

David Katz, MD, MPH, FACPM, FACP, Director of Yale University's Prevention Research Center

Remember that modern-day food environment of ours with the 24/7 availability of food anytime and anywhere? The processed aspect of highly processed food products enables this food environment along with the omnipresence of eating opportunities and their seemingly endless shelf life.

The cheap and easy way to recognize a processed food is to ask yourself: will I find this food occurring in this same condition out in

Want to Apply
Permaculture
ON YOUR PROPERTY NOW?

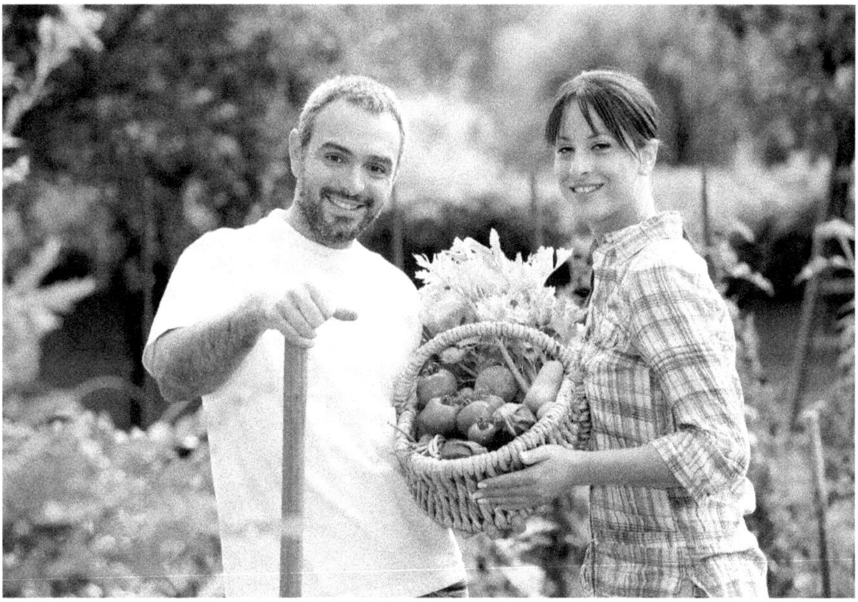

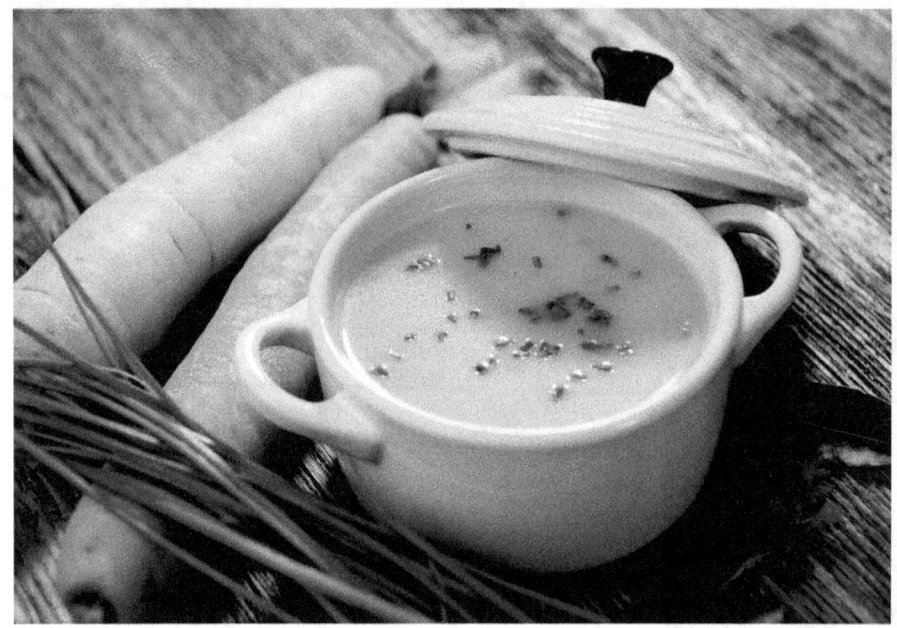

nature? For example, there is no such thing as a tree of Froot Loops or Hot Pockets. You will not find the Bologna Barn at your local farm with little Bolognas grazing in the pasture. Joking aside, this becomes a surprisingly accurate shorthand for identifying processed versus whole foods.

By contrast, whole plant-based foods are recognizable out in nature: even our children can point out an apple tree, pull a carrot from the ground, or identify beans growing on a bush or vine.

The processing of our food really occurs along a spectrum. Returning to the mythical Froot Loop tree for a moment, this well-known breakfast cereal is an example of a *highly processed food*. You have to read its ingredient label pretty closely and decipher the long-winded names of many manufactured additives in order to understand the raw materials required to make a single box of Froot Loops.

Regenerative Leadership Institute
create a meaningful life doing what you love

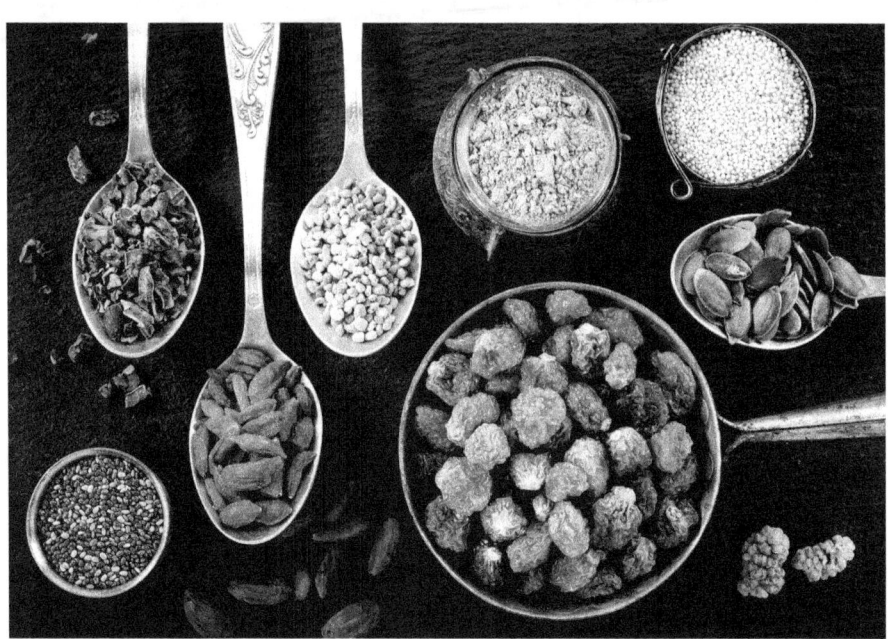

So, what about applesauce? Using our shorthand test, you know you can walk onto a farm and find apples, but it won't look like applesauce. That's because store-bought applesauce is *lightly processed*: it still retains a lot of what it has in its original state, but it has been ground up, which is one method of processing. You can still imagine how it was made from whole, fresh apples, though. If the ingredients label only has one ingredient, apples, then you have your answer: the only raw material required to make that jar of applesauce was apples.

The more highly processed a food, the more likely it was stripped of nutrients – such as vitamins, fiber, and minerals – and the more likely it was packaged with unnecessary and sometimes unhealthy additions. Packaged food companies often include such additives as sugar, salt, artificial colorings and flavors, and certain unhealthy fats to extend shelf life and/or enhance appearance and flavor of the food product, not to benefit our health.

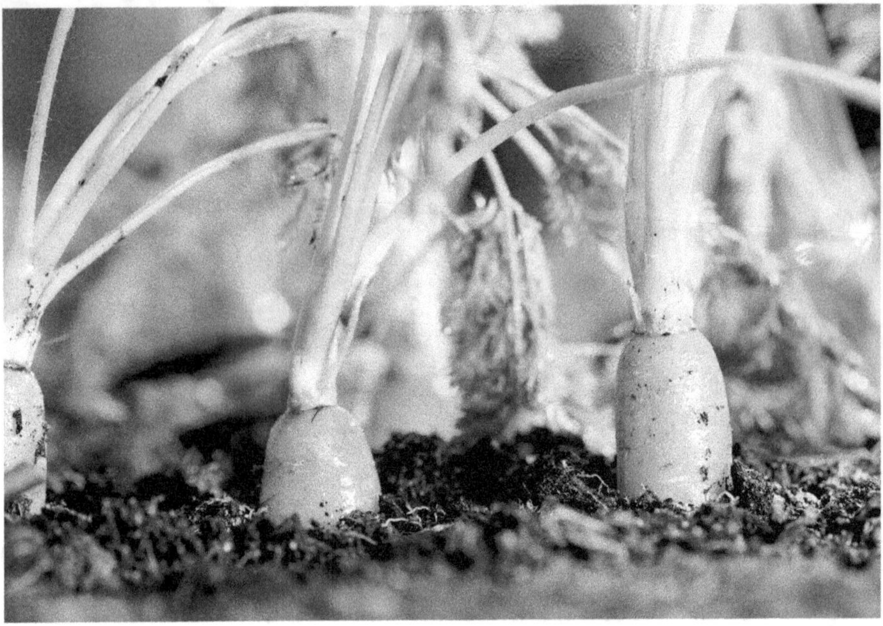

The closer you can get to food in its whole and intact form, the more you benefit from high-quality nutrition, and the more you avoid unhealthy additives.

From Animal Foods to Plant Foods

"It's not just about taking off the pounds; it really is about improving the quality of the fuel your body runs on."

David Katz, MD, MPH, FACPM, FACP, Director of Yale University's Prevention Research Center

Animal foods and plant foods are exactly what they sound like. Animal foods are derived from an animal, and plant foods originate from a plant. Animal foods include milk, cheese, all dairy, meats, processed meats like bologna and sausage, fish, and eggs. Plant foods include fruits, vegetables, legumes, grains, herbs and spices, sea vegetables like nori , kombu and dulse, fungi (mushrooms), nuts, and seeds. ·

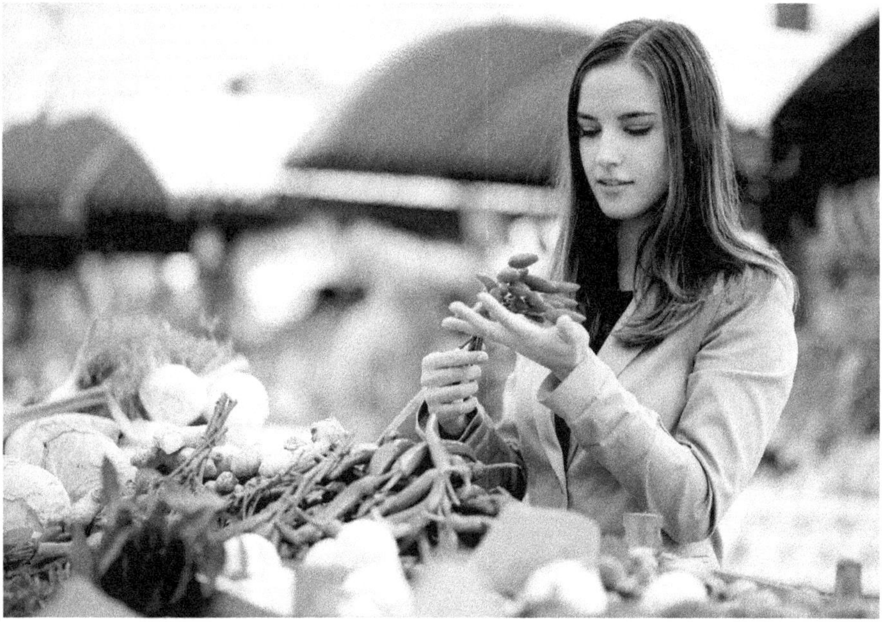

Phytonutrients are chemicals unique to plants that benefit our health in many ways – there are thousands of them, many of which are still being studied. Phytonutrients are a relatively new and exciting frontier in nutrition science research. Despite the hype surrounding the latest food to be deemed *superfood*, the discovery of a new phytonutrient is often responsible for these labels.

In the monumental 20-year China Study, and book by the same name published in 2005, Dr. T. Colin Campbell found that rates of a variety of cancers correlated with the introduction and increasing volume of animal-based foods in the dietary patterns of numerous populations in China. His and other research have also provided strong evidence for the ability of plant-based eating to reduce cholesterol and sometimes reverse evidence of severe cardiovascular disease.

While animal-based foods often possess more concentrated protein by weight, plant-based foods outperform them as fiber-rich (animal foods

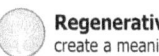

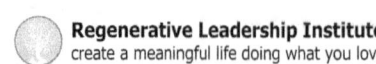

have none), cholesterol-free (plant foods have none), and nutrient-dense (more vitamins, minerals, and phytonutrients per calorie) choices. In fact, dark leafy greens always top the list of most calorically efficient foods evaluated in terms of the nutrients we get in return.

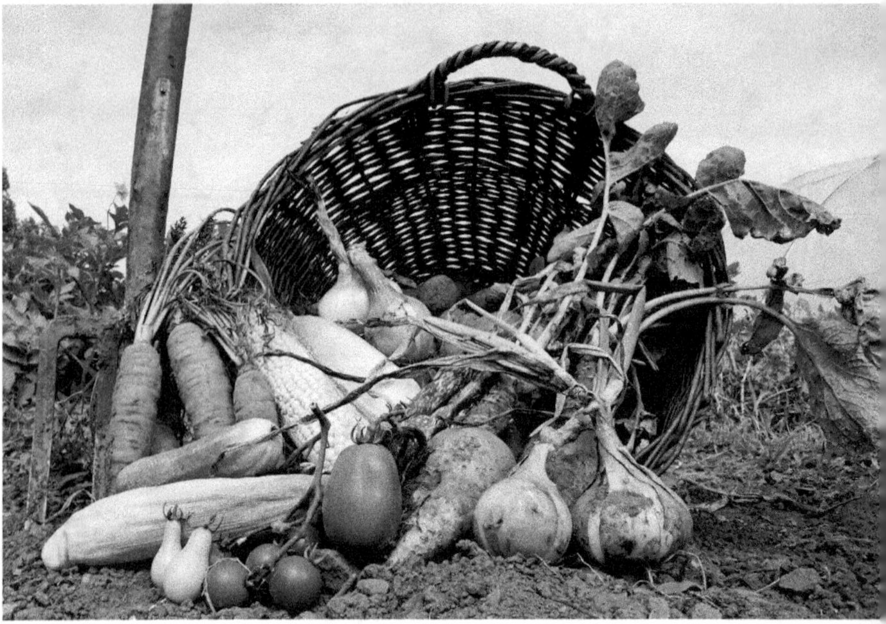

Throughout this transition, we will encourage and show you how to make more and more food choices from the plant world.

From Quantity to Quality

"Food is the most intimate thing you can buy...Unlike clothes and shoes that dress the outside, food goes into your body and builds who you become."

– Ani Phyo, cookbook author, speaker, and raw foods expert

If you have ever set out to lose weight in the past, and that involved diligently counting calories or worrying over portion sizes, then you are

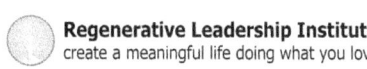

in for a real treat. As if the high nutrient density of whole plant-based foods weren't great enough, they bring another advantage to the table: low calorie density. It typically takes a greater volume of plant foods to arrive at 100 calories than for animal foods. Compare 207 calories in one 4-ounce serving of beef sirloin steak with 40 calories in one 4-ounce serving of broccoli, for example. The fiber in broccoli also contributes to feeling more full or satisfied, whereas the steak has zero fiber.

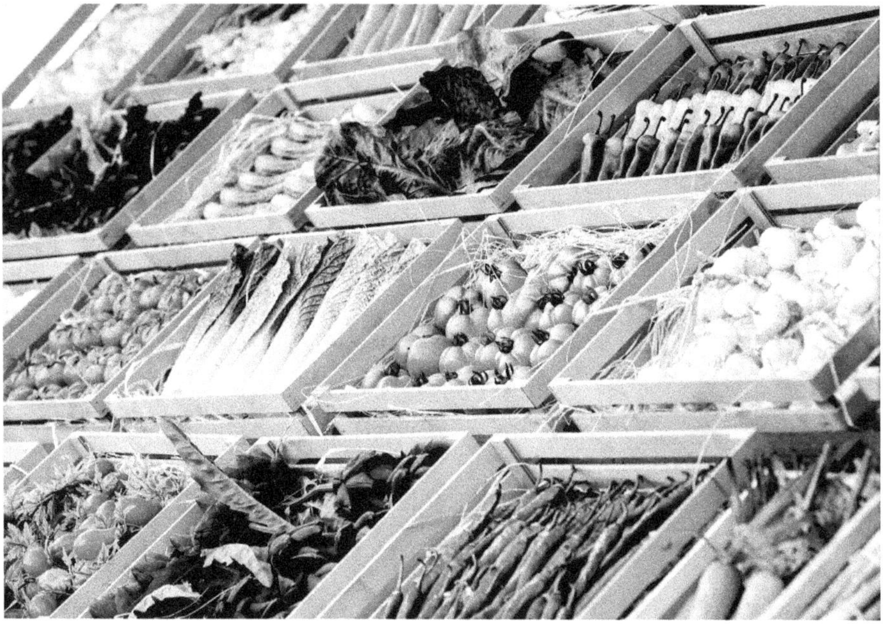

By enhancing the quality of your food, you really up your intake of *micronutrients* – vitamins, minerals, and phytonutrients. Why are micronutrients so important? We all know that we need enough of the macronutrients – carbohydrates, proteins, and fats – for our bodies to carry out all the amazing functions they perform on a daily basis. But, did you know that micronutrients often act as *cofactors* in those very functions? A cofactor is a substance that plays a supporting role but is absolutely necessary for that function to occur. It may not get the fancy title or the media spotlight, but we need it just as much as the leading actor for the show to go on.

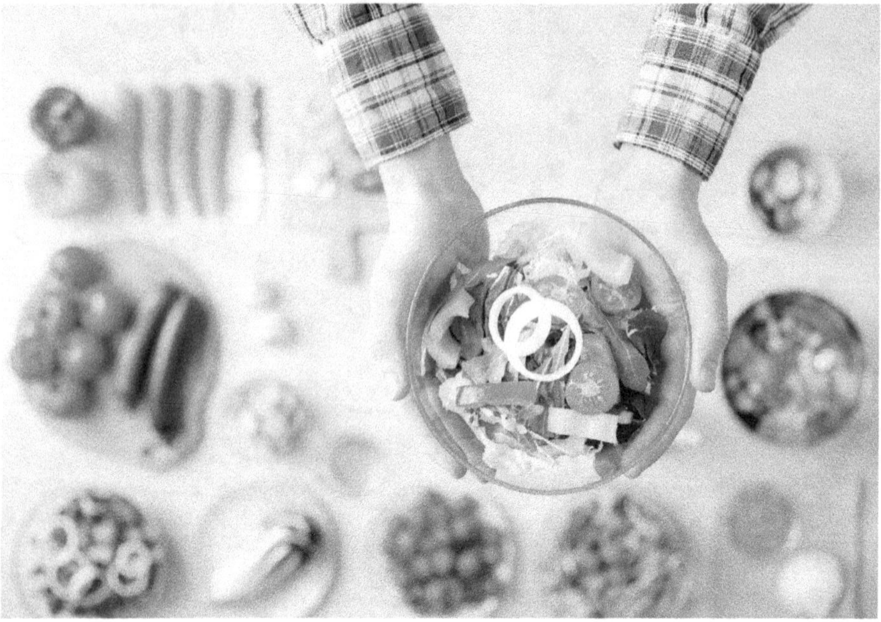

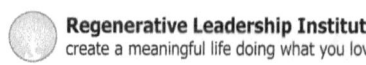

Micronutrients are really the underestimated, underappreciated little guys who keep the machine humming. While the amount of vitamins and minerals we absorb and need from our food is typically very small compared to macronutrients (hence "macro" and "micro"), we still very much rely on their presence throughout the body. Deficiencies in some of the most important vitamins and minerals can also really interfere with processes and dangerously impede certain functions altogether.

A whole, plant-based approach to eating ensures a higher micronutrient intake than any plate of food possible on the average S.A.D. because you are eating directly from the source! Take one example of dairy milk: we celebrate cow's milk for its high calcium content, yet have we ever stopped to consider how or why so much calcium ends up in the milk to begin with? The calcium is not inherent to the cow's milk per se. Instead, the cow's intake of calcium-rich greens and other plants causes the cow's milk to contain calcium.

Regenerative Leadership Institute
create a meaningful life doing what you love

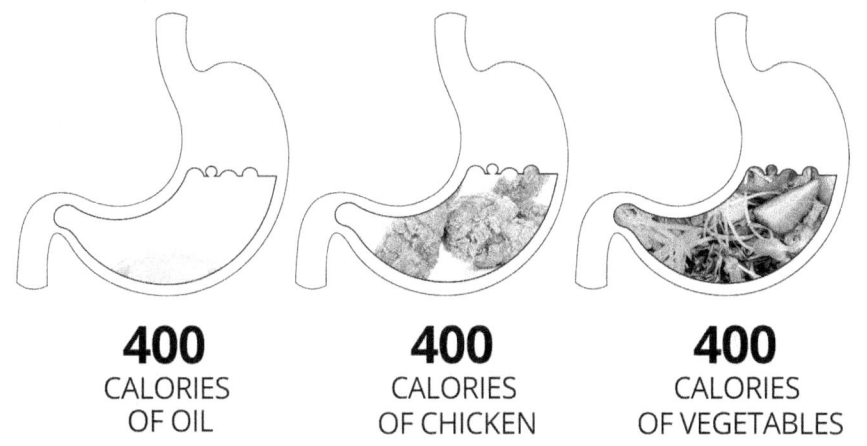

400
CALORIES
OF OIL

400
CALORIES
OF CHICKEN

400
CALORIES
OF VEGETABLES

Why not go directly to the source for your calcium, skipping the unnecessary saturated fat, cholesterol, and hormones?

Vegetables, nuts, and seeds are among the most calcium-rich foods we can eat. Despite some claims to the contrary, an increasing body of research suggests that the bioavailability (or, the ease with which our body absorbs calcium from this source) of calcium from plant foods is just as high if not higher in some cases than from dairy. Bok choy, kale, sesame seeds, watercress, kidney beans, almonds, and figs are just a few.

We encourage you to take this opportunity to reexamine your food choices in terms of quality, not quantity. Even though the average crash diet involves a serious reduction in calories and portion sizes, and even though leaders in the food industry and government frequently prescribe an "exercise more, eat-less approach" to lose weight, we instead urge you to identify foods that offer your body the highest quality of nutrition possible. If you are new to choosing whole plant-based foods, your choices are likely to have lower calorie density and higher nutrient density than ever before, and you won't have to fret over portion sizes.

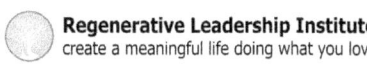

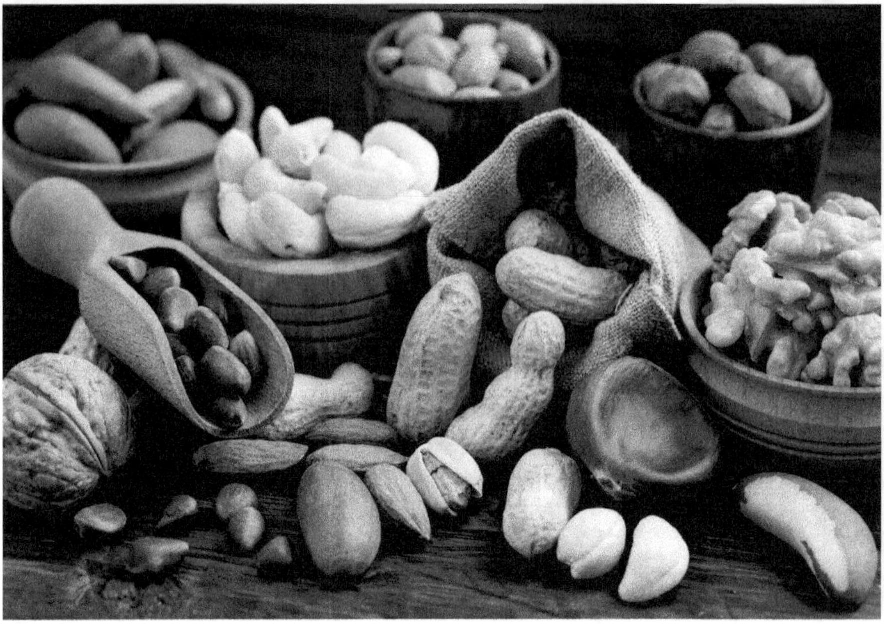

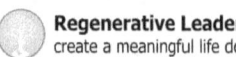

From Mindless Eating to Mindful Eating

"Eat, drink and be mindful."

Susan Albers, Psy.D., eating psychology expert

With 20% (or even more since that 2008 figure) of meals eaten in cars and more foods specifically designed to be eaten on the go with one hand, many of us eat while we do something else. Have you ever been eating something and then looked down at the plate or wrapper and suddenly realized you had finished it without remembering that you did? Many of us have this experience, and our contemporary food environment encourages it.

Eating more mindfully, connecting with the signals your body sends, and noticing how and when your body responds to what can provide both great motivation and great results in your quest to enhance your vitality and lose weight.

Regenerative Leadership Institute
create a meaningful life doing what you love

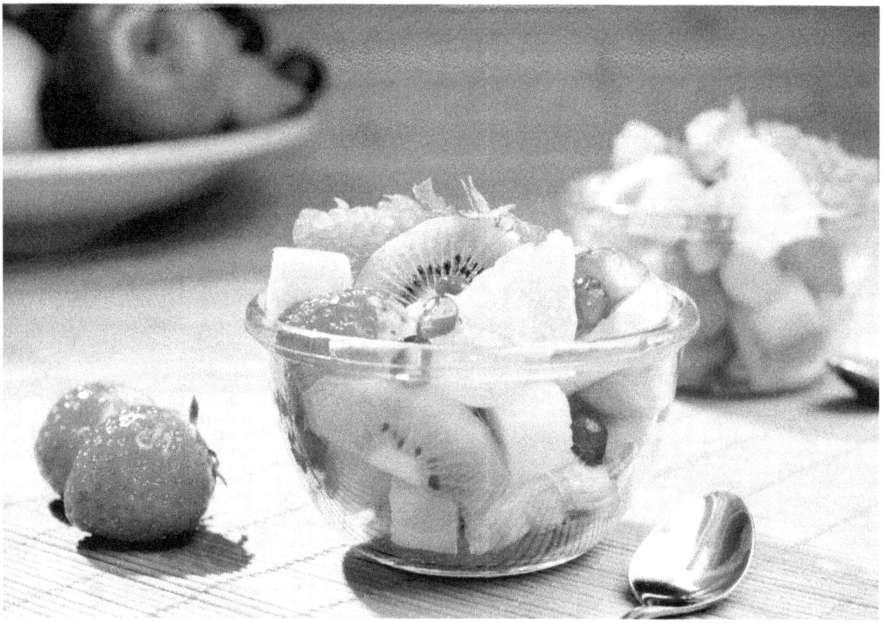

Do this at your next meal: chew a single bite of food at least 50 times before swallowing. You will likely need to focus and count to be sure you chewed at least 50 times. This is challenging and eye-opening for most people who try it! You may notice tastes and textures you never before noticed in a familiar food, or you may realize your current chewing habits are a small fraction of the 50 times you do in this exercise. Depending on what you are eating, you may also notice that your food tastes sweeter than ever before: we have enzymes in our saliva that begin to digest complex carbohydrates into its sweeter-tasting building blocks right away as we chew. If you swallow your bites whole or after only a couple bites, you may never arrive at this sweet taste. This process has evolved in alignment with our biological needs, too. This process facilitates absorption of key nutrients at the very first step of our digestive tract, our mouths! Whatever you notice, it will open your eyes to a process that usually occurs under the radar and outside of our awareness, although it is a process that happens many, many times throughout the day!

Regenerative Leadership Institute
create a meaningful life doing what you love

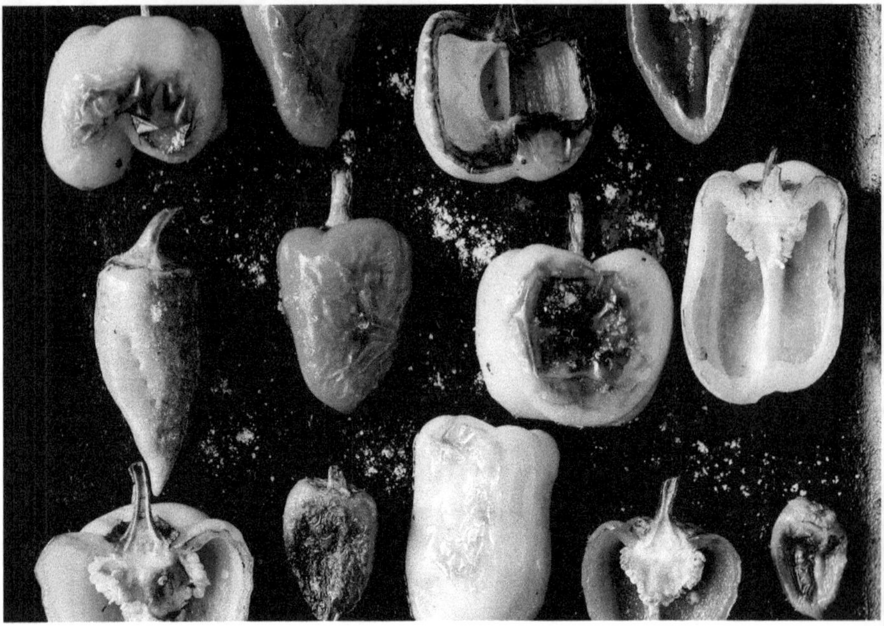

Maybe you'll notice the taste of your food more. Maybe you'll slow down in ways that enhance your body's nutrient absorption and gives your body more time to realize you are full to avoid overeating and digestive discomfort. Maybe you'll notice undesirable side effects for the first time from one of the foods in your daily routine. The journey of mindfulness in eating is always evolving and is different for each of us. There is no "wrong" place to be on this path. It is a continuous practice of noticing, optimizing, recalibrating, and experimenting.

Another way to approach mindfulness in your meals is to notice the environment and the company you keep at mealtimes. You are sure to notice some habits and routines that already work well for you, and perhaps some others that don't support your health and wellness goals. Do you eat differently at different times of day? Do you make different choices after a restful night of sleep or a stressful work day? Do you order differently when you're out with a crowd of good friends versus a business meeting versus a family dinner when you know your kids are watching?

Regenerative Leadership Institute
create a meaningful life doing what you love

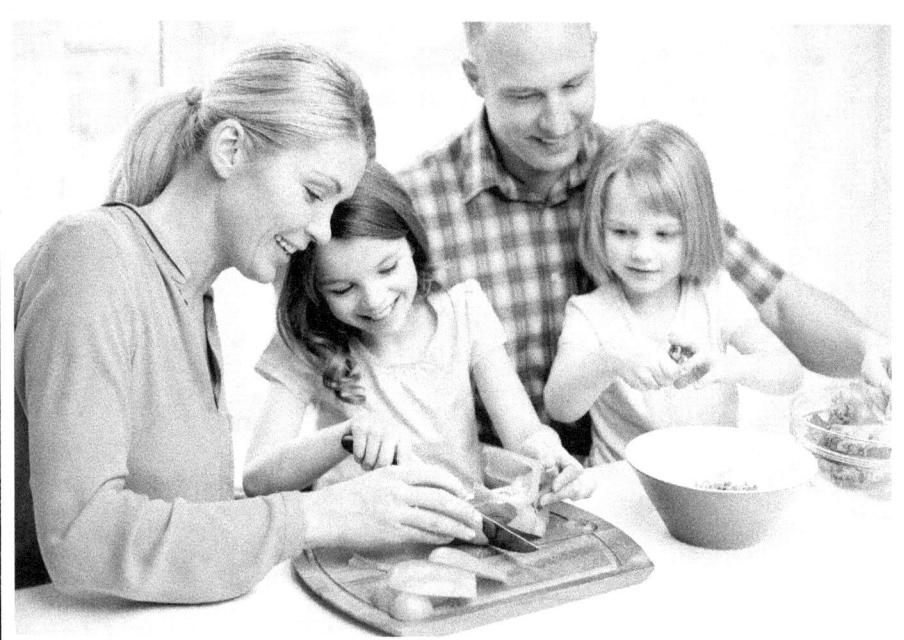

Think of the two healthiest friends or loved ones in your life: how often do you eat with them? Do you know whether your food choices, pace of eating, or anything else is different when you eat with them versus other people in your life? Are you aware of anyone who might be a negative influence on your eating habits, someone with whom you behave differently when it comes to how much you eat or what you decide to order when dining out, or who judges you or makes you uncomfortable about your food choices?

Eating with others is an irreplaceable element of cultures around the world and the everyday lives and routines of many of us. Eating with others can also be very distracting if we are currently making efforts to observe and change our eating habits in any way! Taking a completely private, undistracted, solo meal on your own once a day, week, or month might help you on this path. Talking openly with your friends and family about what you're up to and how they can support you on your journey to a healthier life may also really help. Simply engaging with these questions and answering them for yourself may lead you to insights and next steps all on their own.

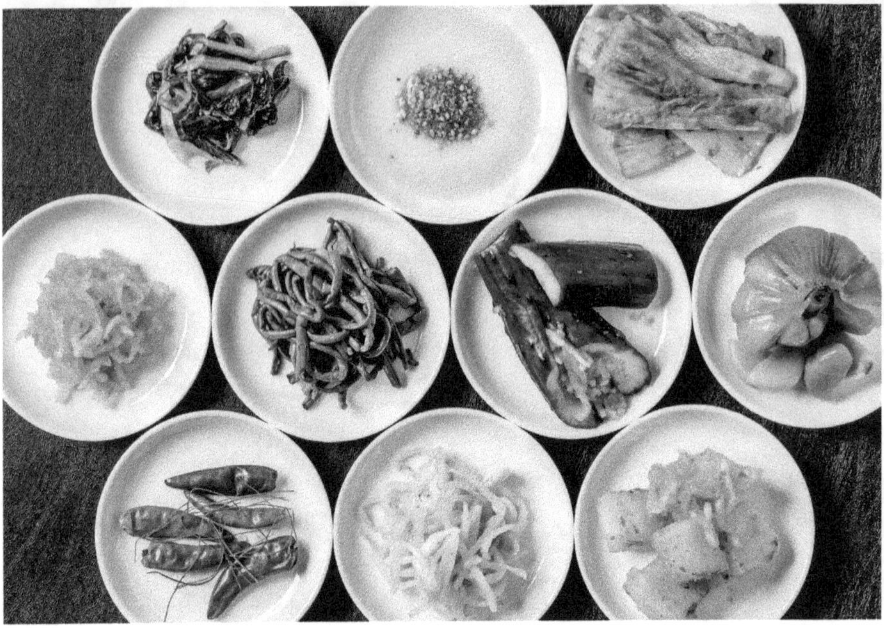

It's All About What You CAN Eat, Not What You Can't

"Successful people are simply those with success habits."

– Brian Tracy, personal development guru

Remember that you chose to pick up this book and reflect on what it would be like to improve your own health and happiness. If someone offers you food that you know will thwart your weight loss effort, don't think or say, "I CAN'T eat that." Our language is very powerful, even the language we choose when we talk to ourselves silently or write in a private journal. Saying that you can't eat something is not the whole truth.

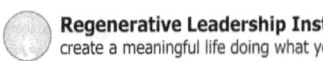

Regenerative Leadership Institute
create a meaningful life doing what you love

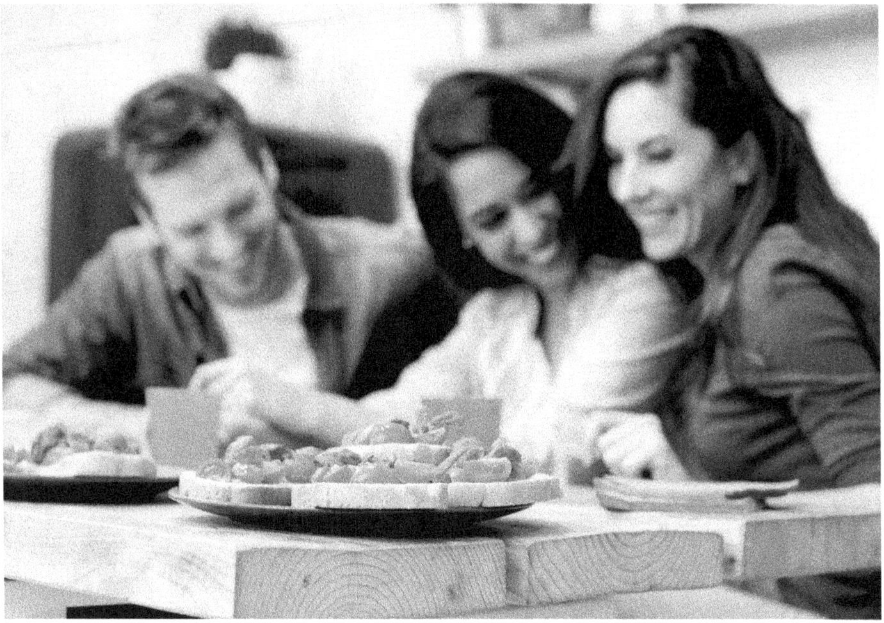

![Three people sitting at a table with food]

You CAN eat it, in fact. No one wired your jaw shut. But you CHOOSE not to eat it. In fact, if it thwarts your ultimate goal and creates frustration for you, *the absolute truth is you DON'T WANT to eat it!* See the difference?

Own your power in this awesome decision you're making for the sake of your vitality and health! We are not the victims of our own decisions.

Hearing the words "I can't" throughout the day, whether spoken to us by someone else or said internally, is discouraging, unmotivating, and disempowering. A mindset that focuses on what you can eat will make the transition infinitely easier since most of us really hate feeling disempowered. Indeed, this is one of the big downsides of deprivation so pervasive in the diet world.

The "I can't" mentality also implies you want it, but that some external force has prevented you from being able to eat it. Again, this is not entirely the case, since you are still in the driver's seat. In the beginning,

 Regenerative Leadership Institute
create a meaningful life doing what you love

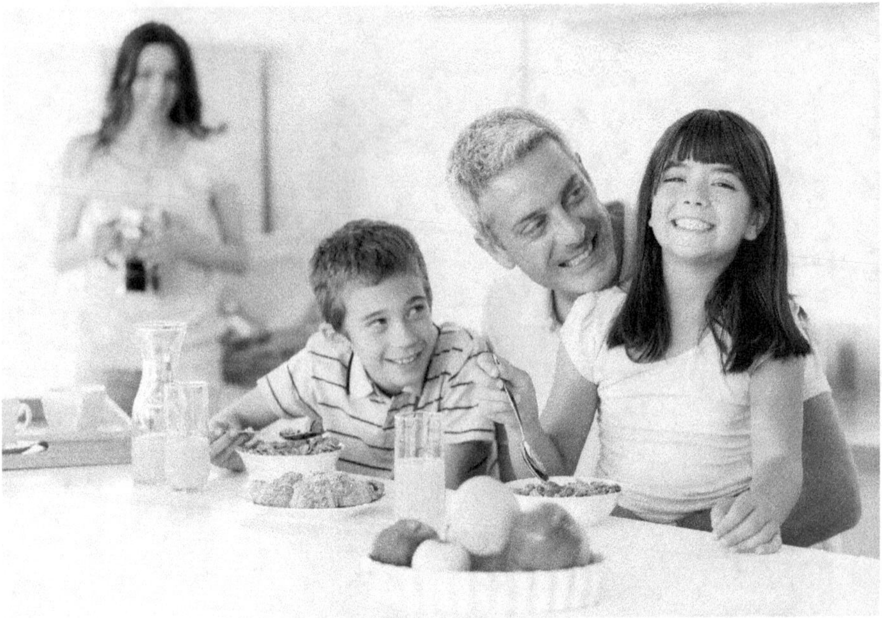

it may be the honest truth that you want the familiar comfort food that you've decided to avoid or cut back on. If this is the case, go ahead and tell yourself and tell others that you want it, and be honest! *And*, you also deserve to hear yourself say why you choose to have less of it or to avoid it altogether in this moment.

Think of it this way: everytime Cheryl says no to a tempting morning doughnut, she is actually saying yes to something else simultaneously. There are two sides to this coin: no to hopping onto a blood sugar rollercoaster for the rest of today, and yes to starting her day off right with a more satisfying breakfast that gives an energy boost to her morning that really lasts! See the difference?

Focus on what is possible, what new realizations and insights will occur, and all that you have to learn and explore. You are boldly setting out to see for yourself what a whole food plant-based lifestyle has to offer and how to make it uniquely work for you. This is an opportunity to

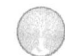

put on your mad scientist lab coat and experiment to see what makes your body feel best and perform best. There are so many whole plant-based foods out there to savor and enjoy, and enhanced vitality and energy and well-being are worth the pursuit!

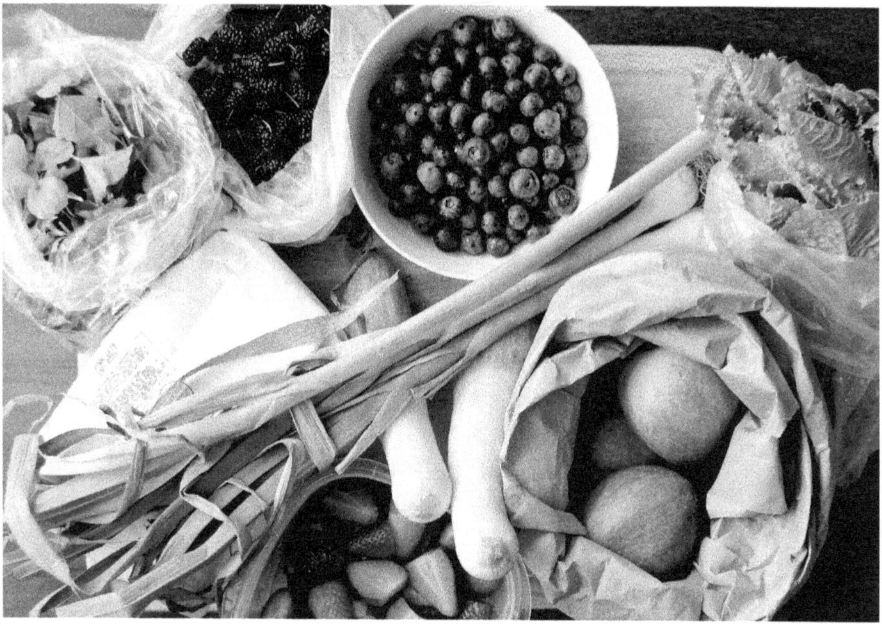

Getting Started

You're jazzed now, right? Ready to launch into our 8-week course to create a healthier life and healthier you?

Before you do, this last section lays an important foundation that you want to have before embarking on any significant lifestyle change. Many people experience challenges in the course of changing eating and lifestyle habits. In those times, we want you to have a steady rock to revisit, like a refueling station where you can renew your commitment, remember what is at stake and why you are doing this, and find your drive again.

Regenerative Leadership Institute
create a meaningful life doing what you love

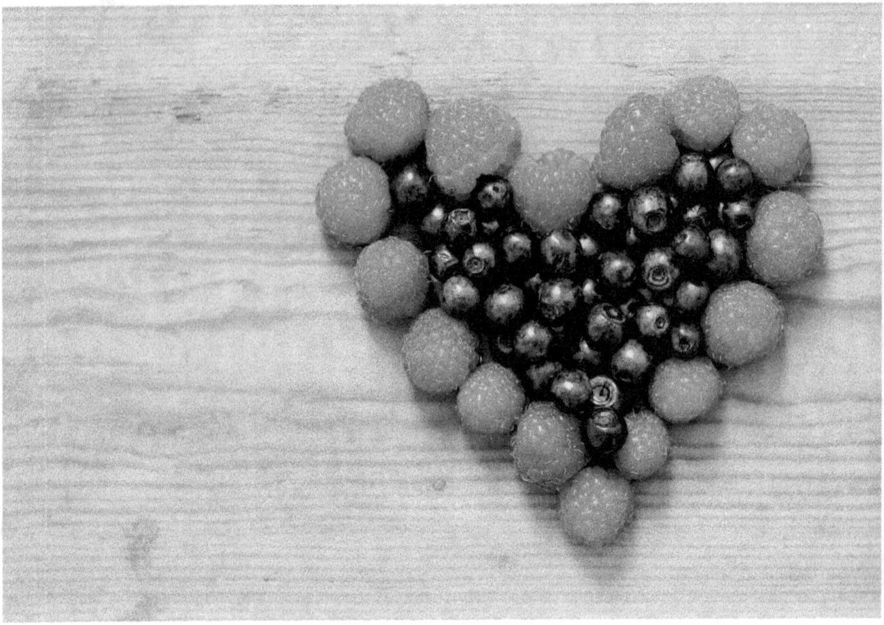

We also want to be sure you get answers to a few commonly asked questions. Plus, we'll give you a special bonus: 5 things you can do right away to start losing weight beyond just changing your food habits. Consider this a warm-up to make the upcoming transition that much easier.

Lastly, we set you up for your launch with some helpful habit change tips and then we'll send you on your way into an amazing 8-week transformation!

Why Are You Doing This? Really?

Don't mistake this for doubting your readiness or commitment. We aren't doing that. Instead, this is an invitation for you to get crystal clear on your own motivation for picking up this book in the first place.

You know the one. The idea or vision or feeling that takes your breath away because every single part of you knows it to be true. The *I-won't-*

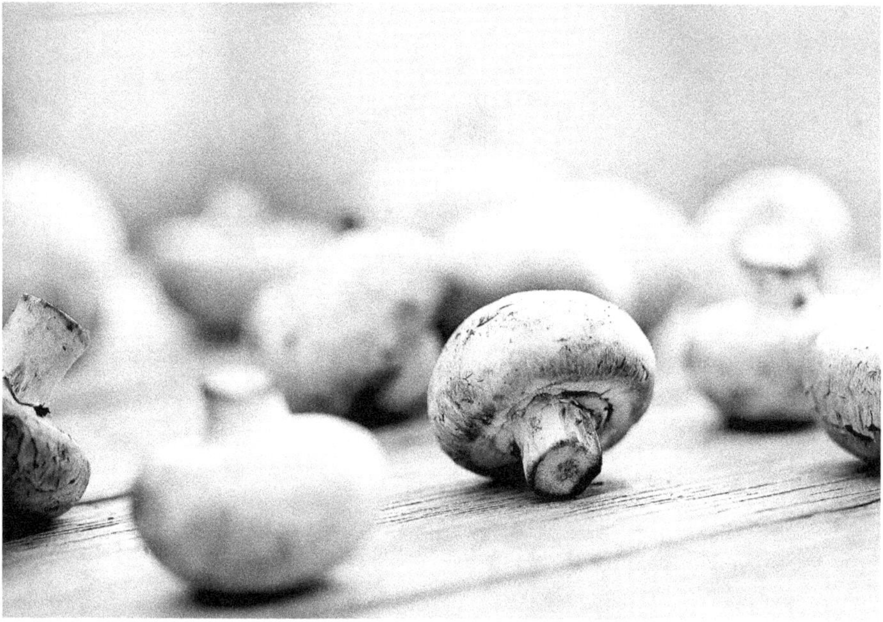

leave-this-dream-or-principle-behind reason that will help you dig deep and remain committed throughout this program. It is normal to have a rough patch or two on the road to new habits as we first break some old habits (we all have them!).

What really moves you to make this change?

What prompts you to set these goals and improve your health at this time in your life? Why now?

Why do you care whether you lose weight or not?

Imagine for a moment that you don't continue forward with us, and whatever it is you seek (more energy, better sleep, less pain or discomfort, easier management of chronic conditions, one or two or all of the above) doesn't happen.

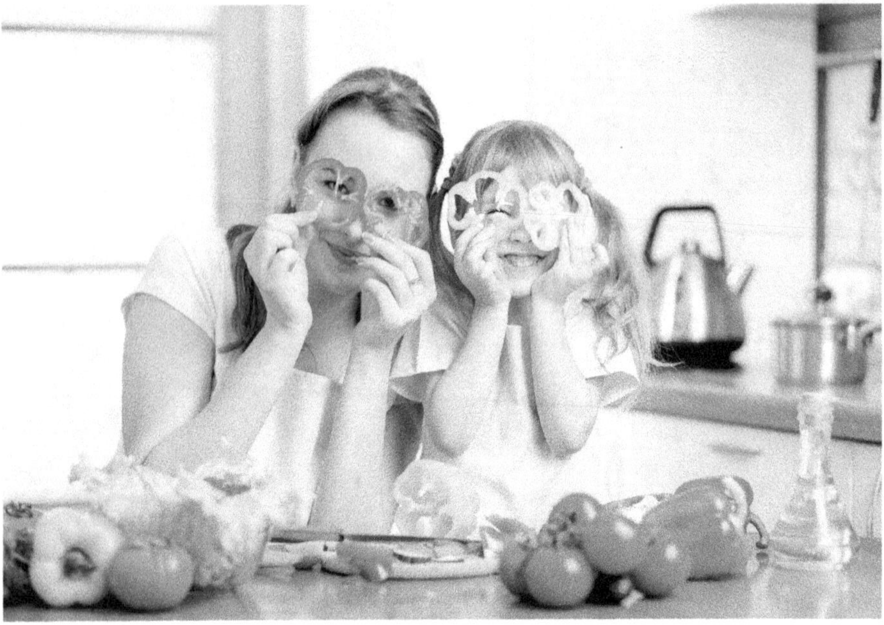

Next, take another moment to imagine that you DO decide to pursue a healthier life during the next 8 weeks in our course. Imagine that what you most want for your health and well-being does come true. In this second scenario, what changes about your life? What will you be able to do that you can't do right now? How will you be able to tell when you are making progress on your goals?

It's easy to get stuck in clichés and platitudes answering these questions. "To be healthier" is a great start, but if you find yourself stopping at that answer, you may benefit from this gentle nudge to go even deeper. You may have to ask yourself a few rounds of "Why?" or "For what?" until you get there, but give it a try.

Then you get into the juicy answers:
To live to see my kid graduate from college.
To feel better when I show up to interview for my promotion so I feel more confident. So I don't die the way my father did.

Regenerative Leadership Institute
create a meaningful life doing what you love

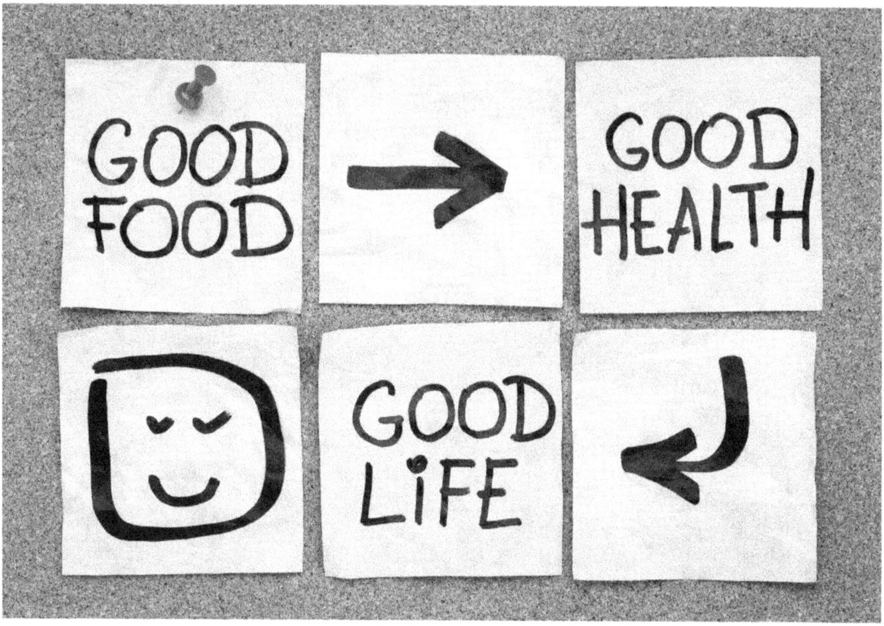

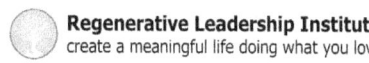

To look my best in wedding pictures that last forever.

See the difference?

You may not relate to any of the answers above, but find the answers that resonate for you. Be as specific as possible in your answer. Get curious and ask yourself "Why?" multiple times if necessary to get there.

We don't know what answer will be most powerful for you. But you do. So, what is it?

Print out this page, take a few minutes of quality time to answer the questions, and put it up somewhere you will see it often.

If the going should feel tough – which, by the way, is totally normal when shifting habits – then you can return to this page and this reason anytime you like. Let it light your fire all over again. This is your secret power source.

Regenerative Leadership Institute
create a meaningful life doing what you love

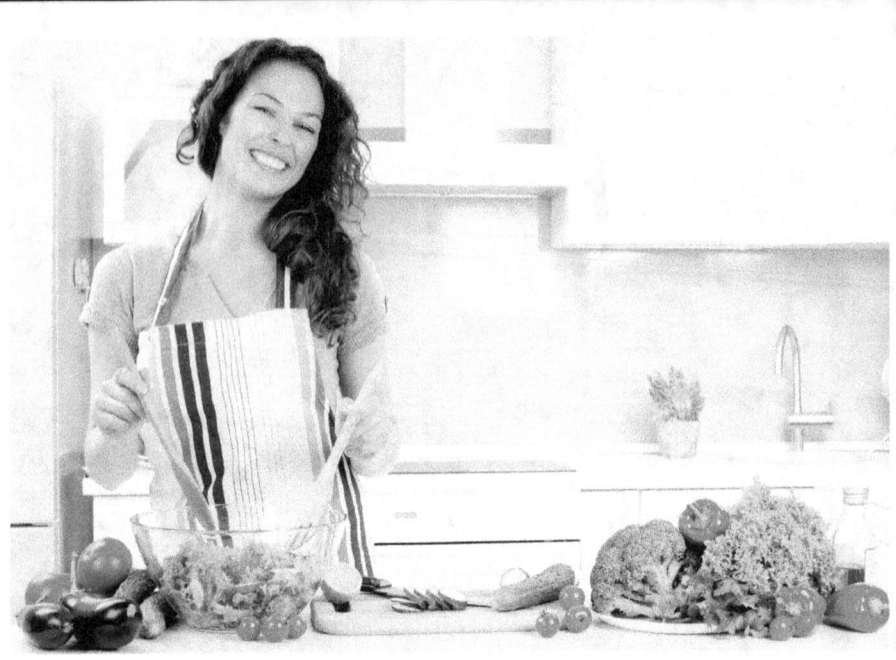

I want a healthier life so that I...

_____

_____

At what point in my life did I feel my very best? What was going on in my life at the time?

_____

_____

Do you believe superior health is possible for you? Do you believe change is possible for you? How do you know?

_____

_____

The most important thing I can do to be healthier is...

_____

_____

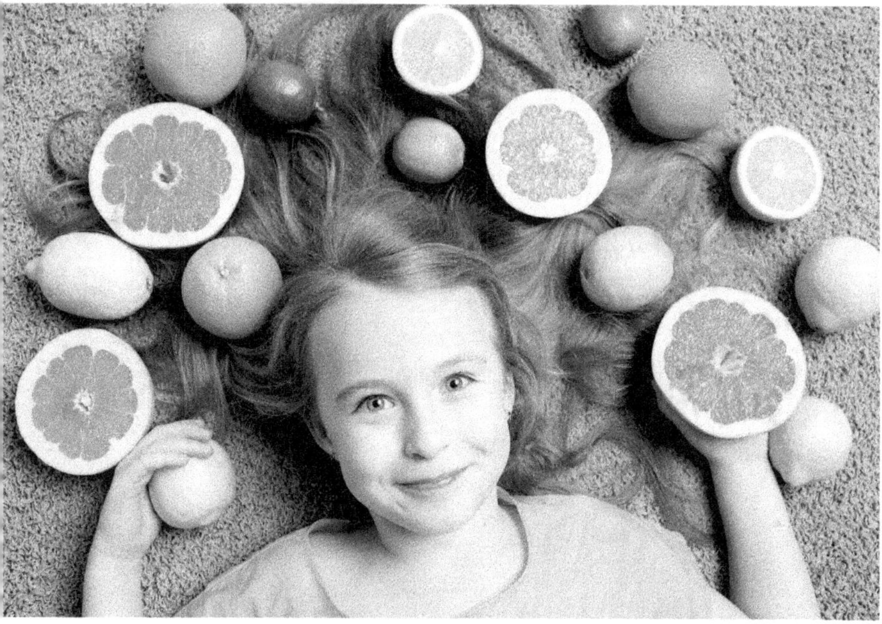

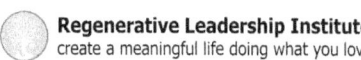

Frequently Asked Questions

Can I really eat this way if I'm just cooking for one? For my whole family? For my children?

Whole food, plant-based meals are every bit as scalable, upward and downward, as any other way to eat. The actual cooking isn't really all that different, so this lifestyle is fortunately relevant for both individuals and families.

The 8-week course concentrates on YOUR experience and supporting YOUR transformation – but don't be surprised when your gradual changes begin to rub off on others! People can actually "catch" habits from each other as if they were a contagious cold: in other words, we influence our peers and social networks with our eating and lifestyle habits, and similarly, we are influenced by the people with which we spend the most time. Your pursuit of a healthier life will positively influence others, sometimes in ways you cannot possibly imagine.

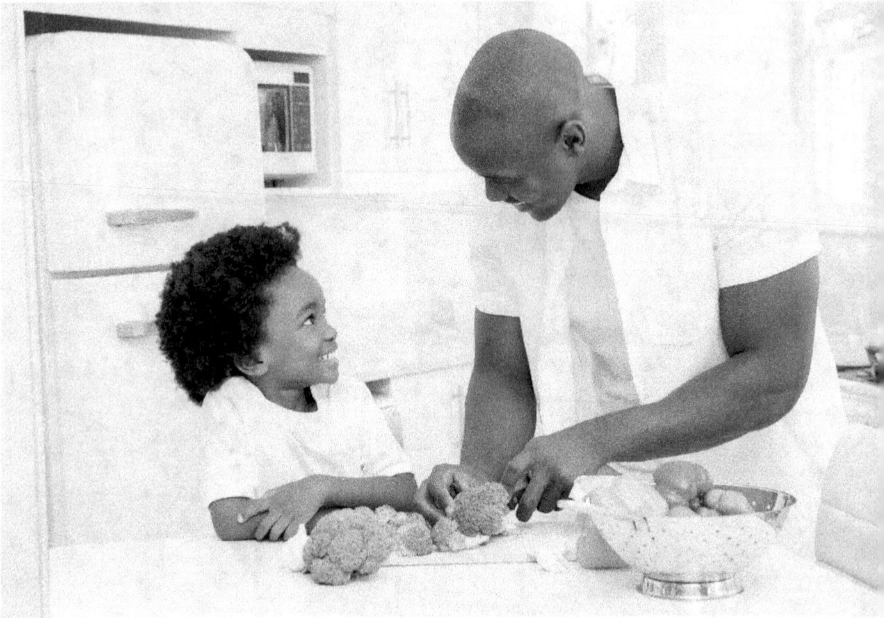

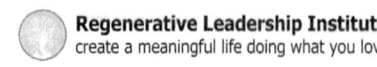

Use this fact to your advantage, and make your transition a social one! The popularity of this eating approach is rapidly growing, and you are never alone on this journey. Finding community during this transition is a great way to line up support for yourself and make new friends. Online recipes, online social media groups and platforms, cookbooks and magazines are easy to find nowadays and cater to whole, plant-based food all the time!

What if I can't imagine life without cheese?

If you can't imagine life without cheese, then don't. There are a variety of nut-based homemade cheese recipes as well as a rapidly growing market of plant-based, non-dairy cheese substitute products available at grocery stores and larger big-box stores like Target, Walmart, and Costco.

What makes dairy cheese so popular? It often has a complex, savory flavor, often called the fifth flavor (after sweet, salty, sour, and bitter), or, *umami*. Parmesan cheese has a particularly high score in terms

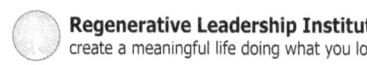

of umami flavor, but it shares that score with another food group: seaweed. Specifically, kombu is one type of seaweed that contains high amounts of an amino acid called glutamate. Kombu is the foundation for Japanese stock soup, which then becomes the base ingredient for a variety of traditional dishes. When our taste receptors detect the presence of glutamate in foods, that is the umami taste.[viii]

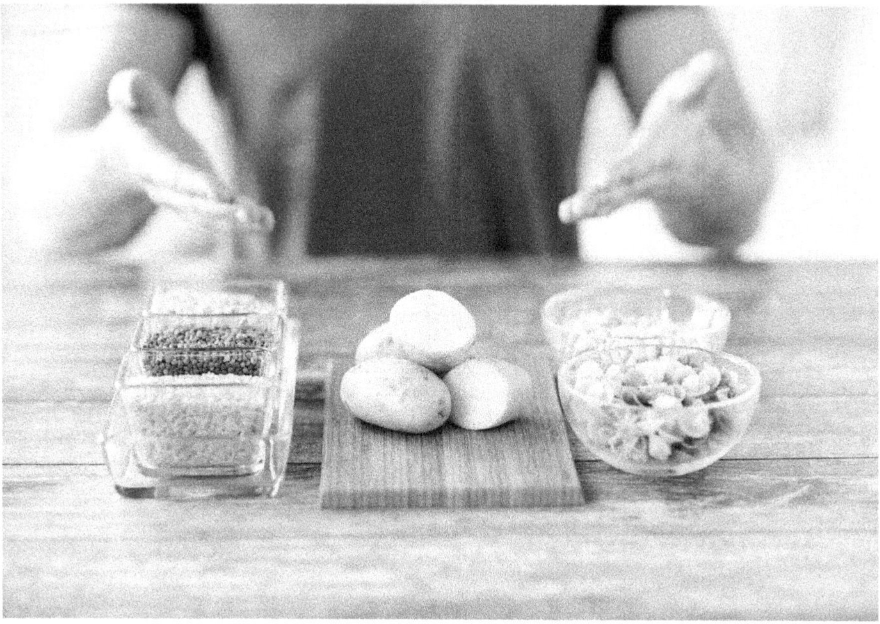

This is really good news, and seaweed is only one example: many plant-based foods boast strong umami flavor owing to their high glutamate content such as fermented foods (kimchi, or fermented Korean vegetables, balsamic vinegar, miso, and soy sauce for instance), tomatoes, shitake and porcini mushrooms, spices like cumin and smoked paprika, and the list goes on.

It is natural to crave the tastes we grew up with. It is natural for your tastebuds to adjust to new flavors, too, and it is easy to trick your tastebuds to enjoy new flavors that are similar to the old favorites.

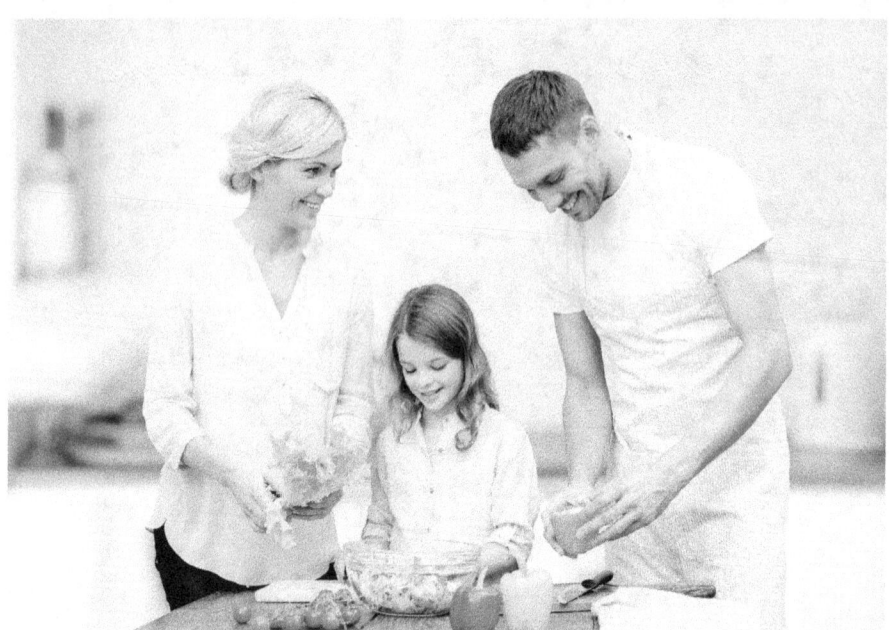

Lastly, often the anticipation is worse than the reality. That goes for many, many things. Remember, you don't have to make all these changes today. And when you are ready to make them, they may not be as difficult as you fear.

These are all great ideas, but what if I want a little more practical help in making the transition?
Our 8-week course is designed to gently guide you through the transition, making only a few changes each week. Two posts a week are devoted to detailed information about the what, how, and why of each week's tips. If you focus on the present week and do your best with the week's recommendations, those small steps really do add up. The general principle throughout the course is that small steps are the way to make big and lasting changes to your health.

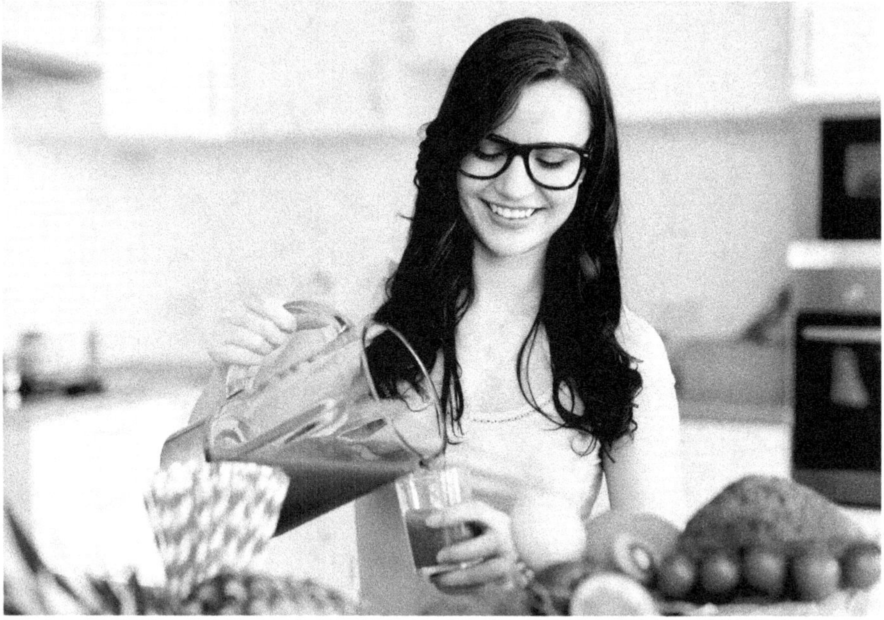

BONUS! Beyond Food: Top 5 Things You Can Do To Start Losing Weight Today

1. Treat your senses. Eating engages many of our senses, flavor is a complex interplay between taste and aroma, and texture even recruits our skeletal muscles when something is crunchy or sticky. No one is telling you to not enjoy your food, certainly not us! Recipes and community around meals are central to cultural identity and families, and a healthy relationship to food includes knowing how to savor and derive pleasure from our food.

At the same time, if you stop for a moment to appreciate the ways in which eating is a very sensory experience, simultaneously you will develop a greater appreciation for other opportunities to engage your senses in ways unrelated to food. If you know you frequently overeat and can't seem to help it, and/or frequently eat for emotional reasons and feel out of control about it, this can be an incredibly valuable insight

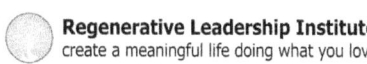

to have. It may reveal underlying causes of cravings and emotional eating habits, and the strategy of treating your senses in ways that go beyond food can be very effective to distract us yet still provide us with the comfort we initially sought from food.

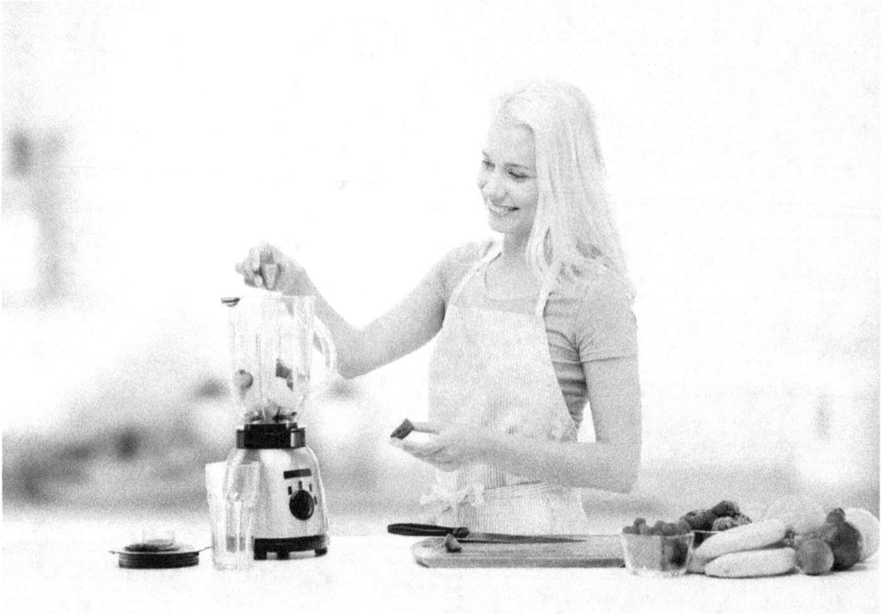

If you don't identify with emotional eating or overeating, but you're interested to learn what you can do to upgrade your health and realize greater well-being, your conscious recognition of eating as a sensory experience is an important one. The more awareness you develop of this concept, the more awareness you develop of the tastes, smells, and textures of your food, and you are bound to discover new-to-you qualities of everyday foods. This is a fun process as well as an useful one as you retrain and transition your tastebuds away from highly processed and artificial food products to whole, plant-based foods. As you tune into your food more deeply and more often, you attune your senses to respond to all stimuli, food and otherwise, in heightened ways. This increases your satisfaction during and after meals, and encourages you to be more mindful and present at mealtimes and the rest of the day!

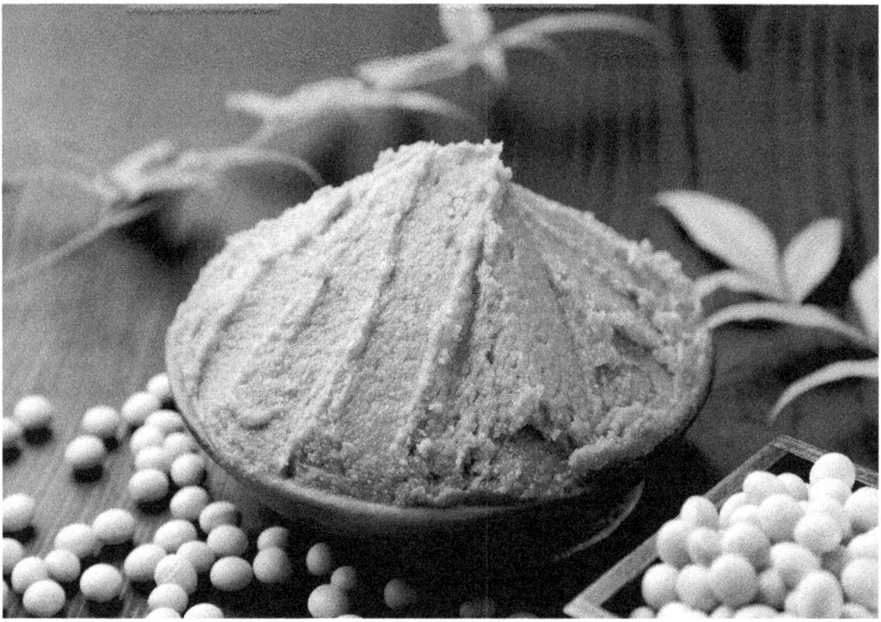

Ready to give this a try? You may be familiar with the "mindfully eating a raisin" exercise – spiritual teachers frequently refer to it as a starting point to understand and practice meditation and mindfulness. For more details on this interesting exercise (including a five-minute audio to guide you!), visit the online home of Jon Kabat-Zinn, Ph.D. of University of Massachusetts Medical School who is credited with this technique among many others.This is Kabat-Zinn's famous exercise (with only a few adaptations of ours) for you to try right now for yourself.

Place a raisin (or other food, doesn't really matter what you choose!) in the palm of your hand. Before you go any further, imagine for a moment that you are an alien life form from another world, and this object in the palm of your hand is entirely unfamiliar and foreign to you. You aren't even sure yet that it is food.

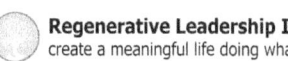

Regenerative Leadership Institute
create a meaningful life doing what you love

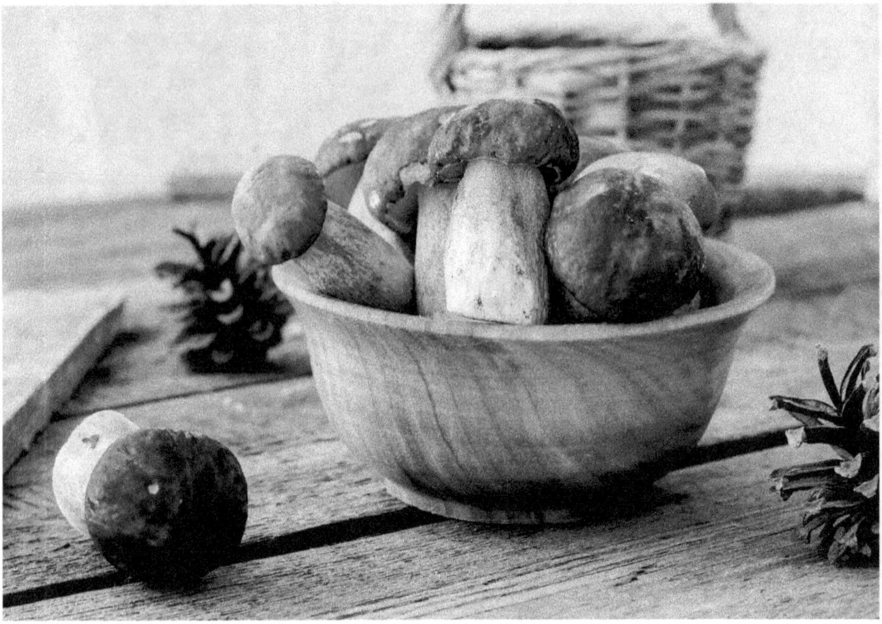

Now, examine this object with new eyes as you systematically engage all of your senses:

- How does it look? What colors do you see? What features on its surface do you notice? Does it reflect light?
- How does it feel in the palm of your hand or with your fingers? Where is it smooth, rough, or bumpy?
- How does it sound? Does it make any sound from the palm of your hand? Does it make any sound when you squish it near your ear?
- How does it smell? How close must it be to your nose in order to detect a smell?
- And finally, how does it taste? Take as long as you possibly can to eat this one raisin – you may need to focus and refocus yourself more than once to slow the natural reflexes our tongue employs once food is in our mouth. Have you ever really noticed before how the tongue methodically moves the food around your mouth, ultimately sending it to the back for swallowing, without you "telling" your tongue to do any of this?

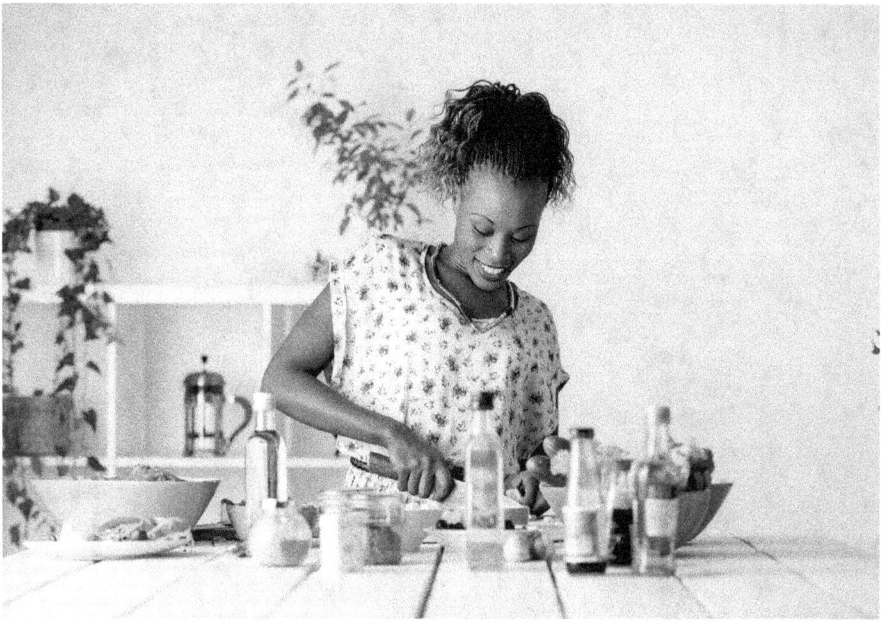

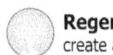

Congratulations! Last thing before you move on from this exercise: take a final moment to reflect on what you noticed during this exercise. Which parts were easy and which parts were not? Did anything surprise you? Did you ever notice yourself resisting to do the exercise at all or frustrated by how slowly the instructions asked you to move? All of this is part of the process, no right or wrong answers, no right or wrong way to experience this exercise. You may even notice that some of your senses are heightened when it comes to other food and other non-edible experiences later in the day as a result of this simple exercise!

Here are some other ways to treat your senses that are useful both for improving your mood, energy, and well-being in the moment as well as providing alternatives to overeating and emotional eating when comfort of a non-edible variety will do the job just as well!

- **Experiment with temperature:** apply a water bottle, hot pack, or washcloth filled with warm water to any part of the body that could

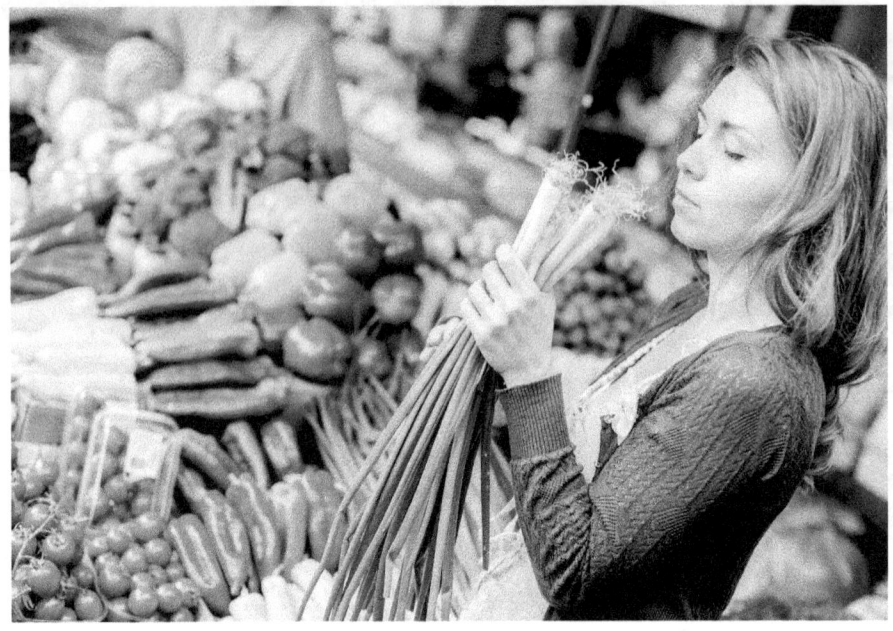

benefit from some comfort. Take a warm bath or shower, or soak your feet in a bathtub of warm water. Many people find warmth more comforting than cold, but depending on the weather, this can all change! Not just for hot days, a cold pack, a water bottle filled with ice water, or a cold-rinsed washcloth can bring great relief to an aching muscle or sore spot, too.

- ***Experiment with light:*** many people enjoy improvements to their mood, energy, and sleep when they intentionally expose themselves to bright indoor light or direct sunlight at strategic times of the day. Direct sunlight is one of the signals that inform our circadian rhythms and internal clock, which have all kinds of effects on our hormones and other biological processes. Exposure to bright light during the daytime can bring immediate comfort and an uplifting boost in that moment, and it may also support more regular sleep times and wake times and higher quality of sleep during the dark hours of the day.

Regenerative Leadership Institute
create a meaningful life doing what you love

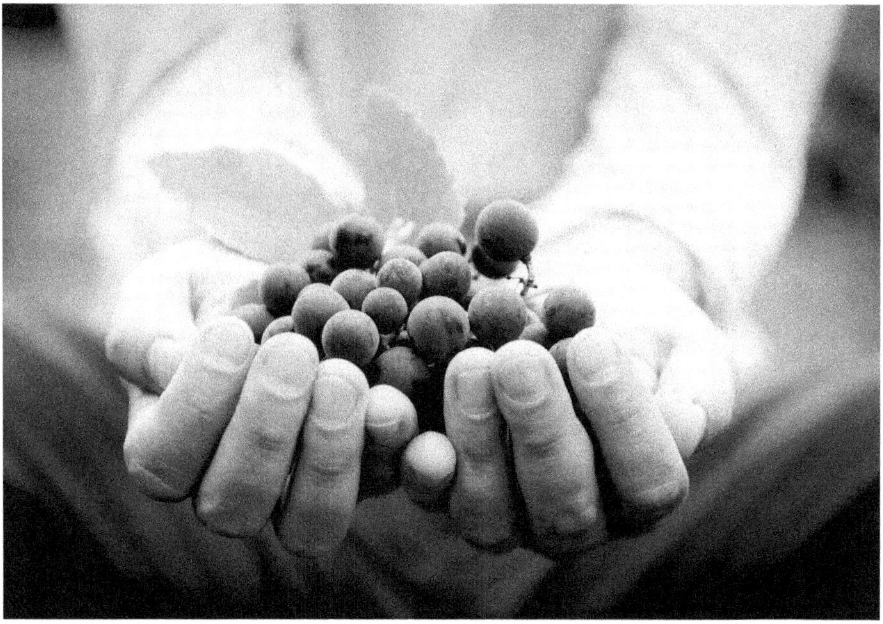

![hands holding grapes]

- ***Experiment with texture.*** The soothing texture of cotton flannel or luxuriously soft microfiber can bring incredible comfort as a towel, blanket, or clothing. Wearing or enveloping ourselves in cozy materials engages our senses and invites us to live in the present moment!

2. *Move more. Today.* If you are reading this too late in the day, or on a day when fitting in a workout is impossible, then you're right – don't bother dashing off to the gym. Instead, find a way to create a 5 or 15-minute activity break sometime before you go to sleep tonight. No fancy equipment, no fancy shoes or outfit, just you moving your body in a natural way to slightly increase your heart rate and get the endorphins flowing. Where can you find an opportunity or excuse to move a bit more than usual?

- take the stairs instead of the elevator
- run after your young children for a few minutes
- park farther from the store entrance

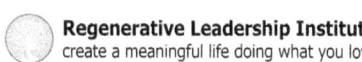

Regenerative Leadership Institute
create a meaningful life doing what you love

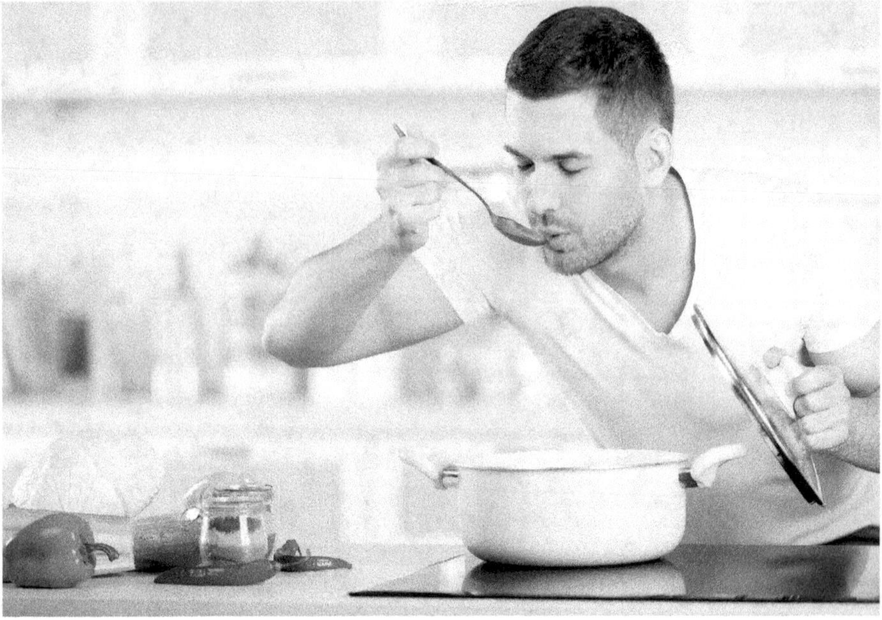

- dance to a playlist of your five favorite songs
- play with your companion animal/s
- take your companion animal/s out for a walk
- vacumming, dusting, carrying laundry or groceries up and down the stairs
- walk around the interior or perimeter of the office building for your business meetings
- walk at a park or around the block when you are on the phone
- turn your social visits into walk-and-talk dates with friends instead of the restaurant or cafe

After reading this list, what other ideas can you think of that naturally appeal to you and feel most realistic to you? They can even be a little scary and new, but something you're curious about and willing to try:

1 _____

2 _____

3 _____

Regenerative Leadership Institute
create a meaningful life doing what you love

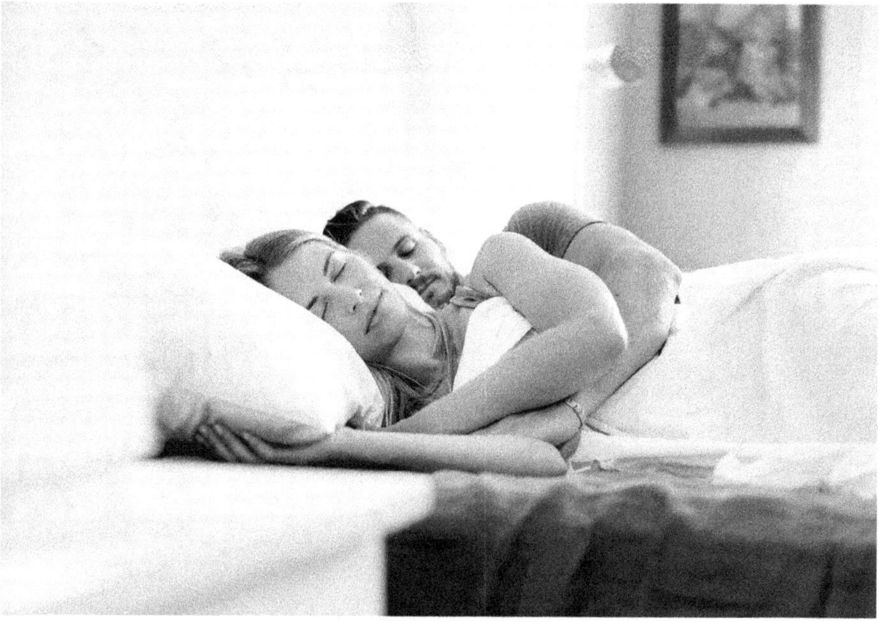

Every time you integrate a bit more movement into your day, you help stoke your metabolic fire and energize yourself!

3. *Get good sleep.* Lack of sleep is a form of stress that cues the body to release a hormone called cortisol. Cortisol plays many important and beneficial roles in our bodies, but chronic sleep deprivation causes chronically high cortisol levels, and that can actually impede weight loss. The nuances in the relationship between cortisol and insulin are still under much investigation, but strong evidence suggests that elevated cortisol can decrease the body's responsiveness to insulin, which increases our chances for developing insulin resistance and other precursors to diabetes. Do the best you can to implement good sleep hygiene in your home and your bedroom, and aim for at least 7 hours of sleep.

It can seem like going without sleep or less sleep gives us those few extra hours we have been looking for to tie up loose ends from work

Regenerative Leadership Institute
create a meaningful life doing what you love

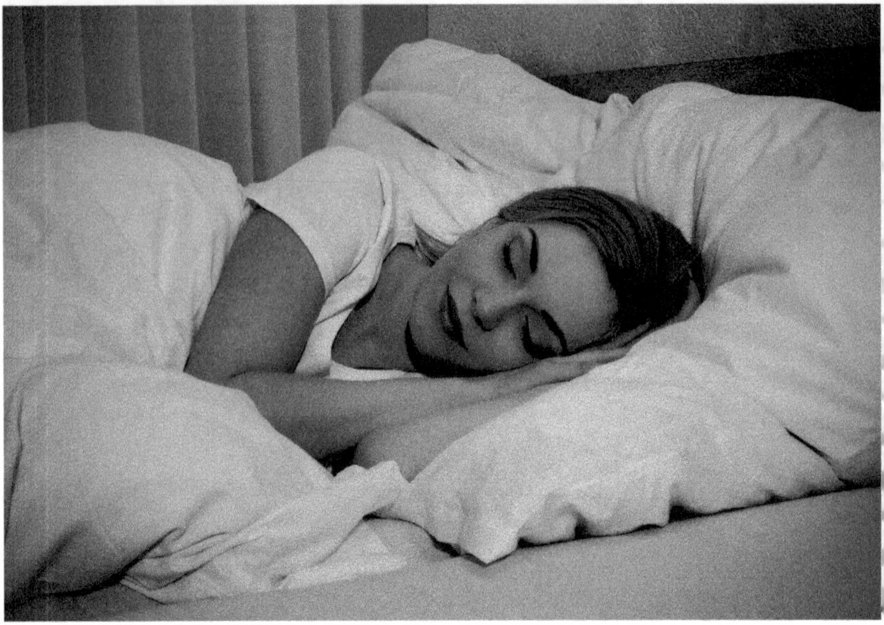

or tackle household chores, for instance. These missed hours of sleep always come at a price, however. As tempting as it can be to postpone sleep, especially when faced with too many things to do, consider this: a solid night of sleep is likely to make you twice as effective in half the time compared with your ability to focus, concentrate, be efficient and physically energetic following a night of sleep deprivation.

When it comes to bedtime, good sleep hygiene translated:
• Use the bed only for sleep or sex
• Avoid electronic screens in bed with you or right before bed
• Keep a regular sleep time and wake time
• Make your sleeping space as dark as possible.

Beyond bedtime, what else can you do to increase your chances of a restful and restorative night's sleep? A few ideas:
• You've likely been told at some point that breathing techniques at bedtime can help the mind and body to relax and allow for sleepiness

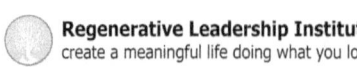

Regenerative Leadership Institute
create a meaningful life doing what you love

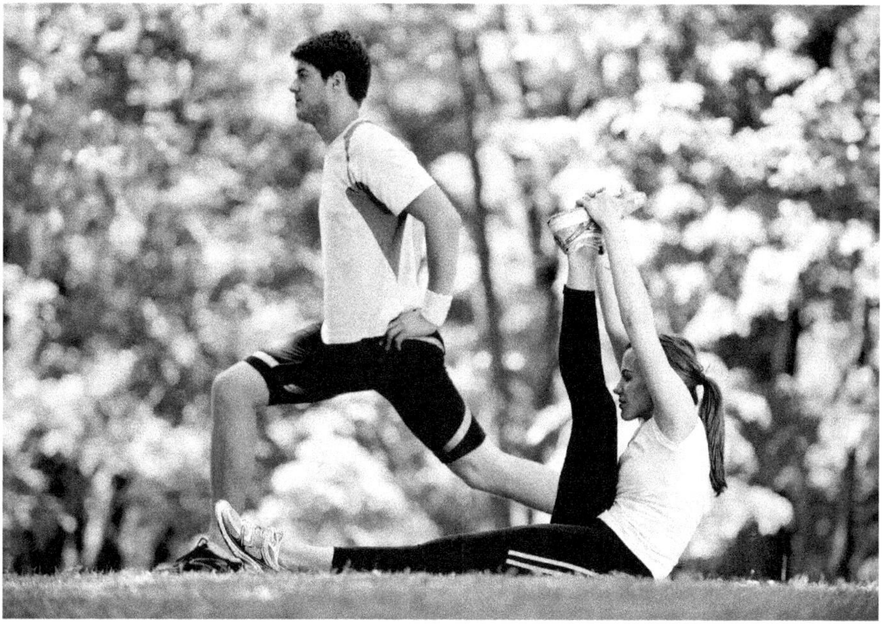

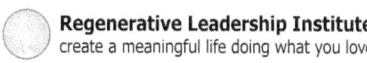

to take over. However, engaging in breathing techniques throughout the day can also help, even if it is hours before your bedtime! When you identify breathing practices that are uniquely effective for you to induce a quiet, calm state, you are essentially training for bedtime. The more you practice deep belly breathing during the day – all it may take is a few cycles when you wake, a cycle before and after meals, and/or a cycle or two during your work breaks, e.g. – the easier it becomes to calm and self-soothe yourself at bedtime (or, when you wake up during the night and want to put yourself back to sleep).

• Exercise is known to be an effective sleep aid. Avoid exercising within a couple hours of your bedtime, since the natural energy boost following physical activity can act as a stimulant for some folks. But otherwise, exercise earlier in the day circulates bodily fluids, regulates healthy hormonal levels, activates stubborn digestion issues like constipation, and more. This can be as simple as gentle stretching or yoga for a few minutes as a morning ritual, or as strenuous as a heart-

Regenerative Leadership Institute
create a meaningful life doing what you love

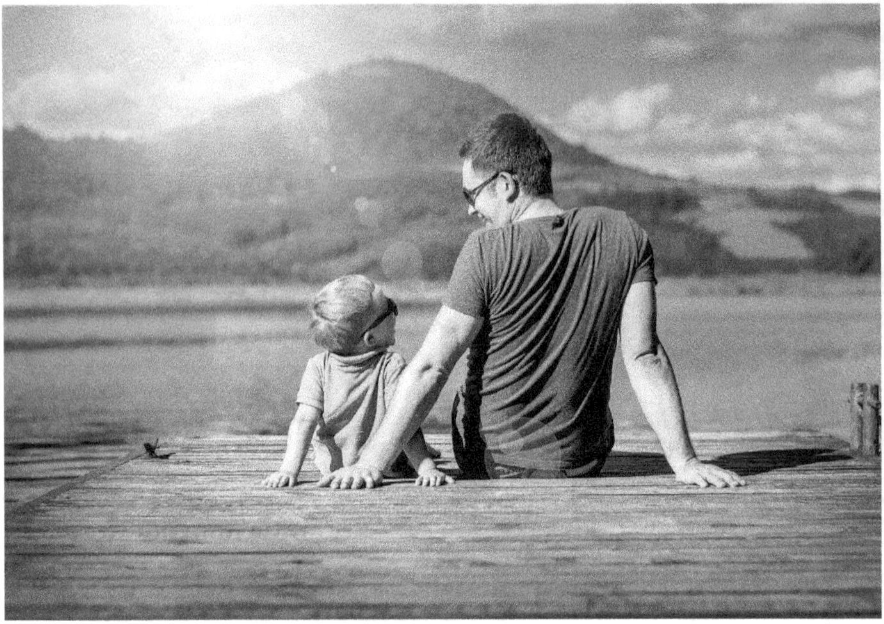

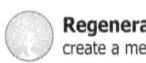

pumping group fitness gym class or fitness video at home. You must experiment and watch for possible connections with the quality of your sleep to find what will uniquely work for you.

• Caffeine is a substance that takes hours for our body to process, and its stimulating effects can be seen several hours following consumption. If you want to sleep better than you do now, if you have trouble falling asleep initially, if you wake up once or more during the night and can't fall back asleep, and if caffeine appears in your daily diet as energy drinks, sodas, coffee or coffee-flavored drinks, you owe it to yourself to experiment with a gradual decrease and even elimination of caffeine for a short time to observe its effects. For many people, this makes a big difference, even though many of us have emotional and comforting associations with our caffeine intake. Tea is usually a more gentle option, although stronger black and green teas do contain some caffeine, albeit less than coffee, so if you switched to tea and the sleeping concerns persist, you might want to avoid all caffeine for a while to allow your body to reset and watch for any differences.

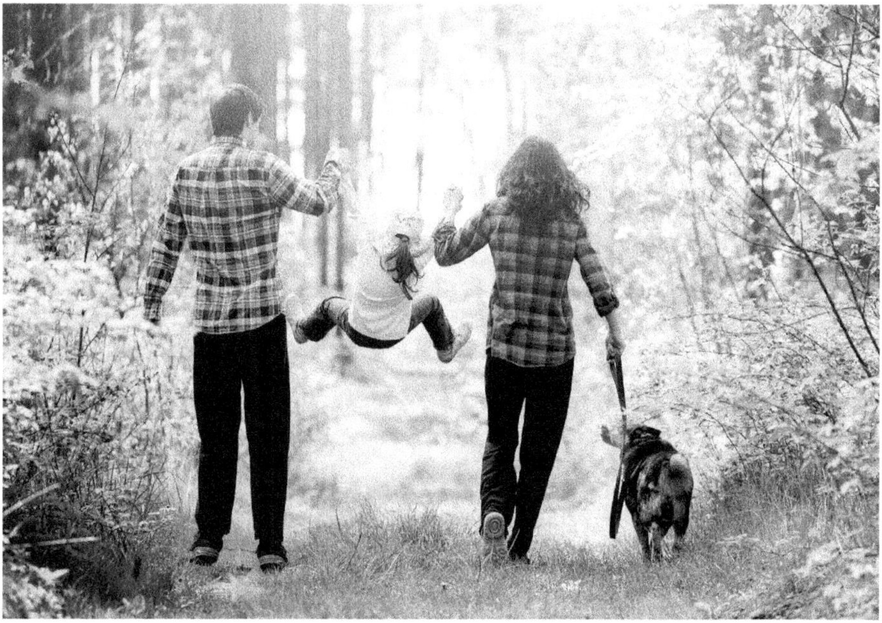

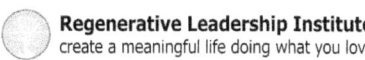

Not enough sleep can interrupt natural circadian rhythms as well as hormonal cycles that together help to signal important cues like hunger and satiety. For all of these reasons, good sleep is really a foundation to increase your energy, lose extra weight, and maintain a healthful weight.

4. *Chill out.* Our bodies respond to various kinds of stress in marvelously complex and effective ways. Yet, our reaction to stress does not easily adapt to the particular nature of that stress. In other words, our bodies do not know the difference between the stress created by a string of sleepless nights, or the stress created by angst over a challenging situation at work, or the stress of being chased by a predator.

The kind of stress that many of us experience these days is chronic – it may even be low grade or not terribly severe, but it is nearly always present because of the increasingly demanding nature of our lives. Such chronic stress triggers the release of cortisol, similarly to how we previously described with respect to sleep.

Regenerative Leadership Institute
create a meaningful life doing what you love

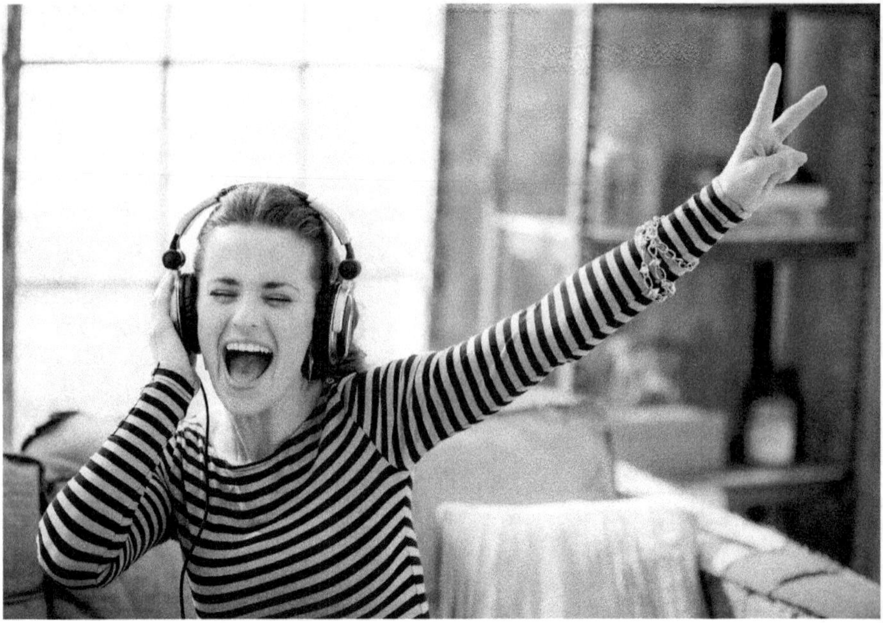

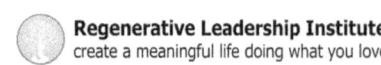

Chronic overexposure to cortisol has damaging consequences for us over the long term, not the least of which is that fat storage is favored during times of stress as a protective mechanism. Great for surviving a famine, not so great for those of us who want to lose extra weight but happen to be stressed out. Finding a way to prioritize rituals and practices that calm your mind and allow you to let go and process your emotions and high stress levels will truly benefit your weight loss goals.

Maybe you will find one new-to-you relaxation idea from this list to try out:
• Chill out to a mellow playlist, your favorite song, or sample music from a genre you know nothing about to try something new
• Follow a guided meditation – you can find online audios or videos to lead you in meditation for as little or as much time as you like, some are as short as 5 minutes! Your place of worship, local community center, local gym or other fitness center, or local yoga and pilates studio may offer free or low-cost guided meditation groups as well if you prefer to do this with others.

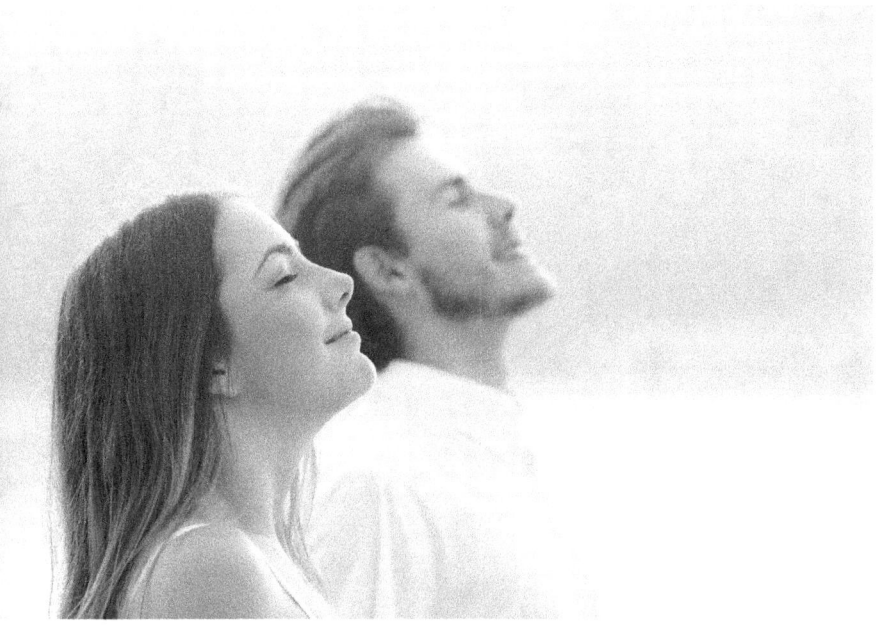

• Snuggle with your companion animals or exchange an extra hug with a loved one

• Self-massage with an exfoliating shower sponge or your fingertips on your scalp, or foot rub

• Warmth is very soothing and relaxing for many people, so try any of these to distract and relax you: a warm washcloth, warm water-filled bottle or other sealed container, or hot pack on your lower belly, neck, back, or laid over your eyes with your lids closed.

• Laugh! Have you ever went searching through your bookshelf, home movies, or an internet search engine with the sole purpose of finding something to make you laugh? Find something new or return to an old favorite that you know makes you laugh out loud, and indulge in it for at least 5 minutes. Just a few minutes of out-loud belly laughter triggers release of feel-good hormones, encourages deep breaths and discourages shallow breathing, and brightens our mood.

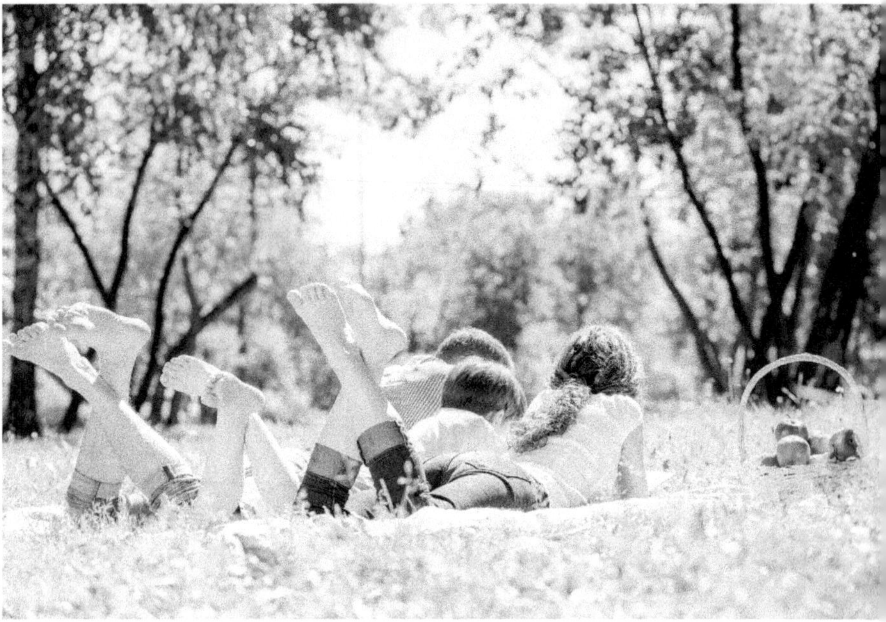

5. *Put on your detective hat.* The simple act of observing ourselves can have a major
impact on our behavior. Set a goal to keep track of something about your eating habits today that you are genuinely curious about. Perhaps:
• How much water you drink
• When and what you snack on in between meals
• How many cups of coffee you drink
• How many servings of fruit and vegetable find their way onto your plate
• When and what you crave

Keep track of your goal in a way that is easy to you – perhaps a simple tally using pen and paper, or something electronic if you prefer. Promise yourself that you won't judge yourself, shame yourself about anything you do or don't do, or exert willpower to do anything differently. Instead, your job is to notice, observe, and record as objectively as possible.

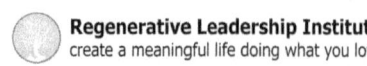

Regenerative Leadership Institute
create a meaningful life doing what you love

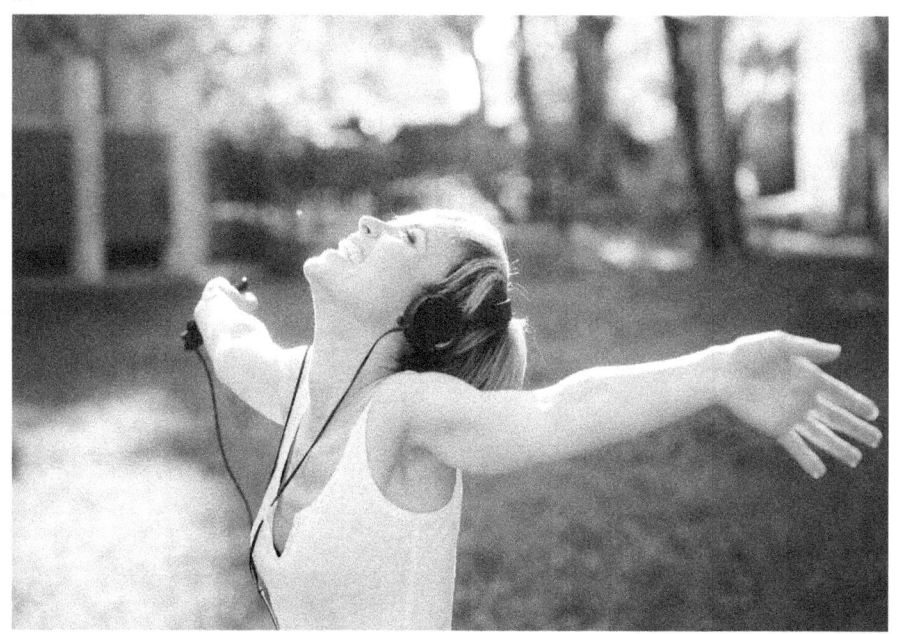

Even though you haven't decided to change anything about what, how, or when you eat, this simple act of self-observation and recording enables your habits to enter your unconscious awareness in sometimes surprising ways, and this experiment also introduces some accountability (albeit internal) where there perhaps was none before.

Better yet, do this for a few days, or even a week, and see what you notice and learn about yourself. This is priceless information that reveals to you what you already do well, what you most want to change about your eating habits, and whether your current habits and choices truly serve you right now or not. After doing an experiment like this, it may suddenly feel much easier to ditch an unhealthy habit or cut back on something that you've previously tried with little success: this may be because you have gained insight into the how and why of this habit, and now that you better understand yourself, you know how to change it and perhaps replace it with something healthier that fulfills the same need. Just one example of the unique insights you gain from doing experiments like this, and all it took was putting on your detective hat, no extreme acts of willpower required.

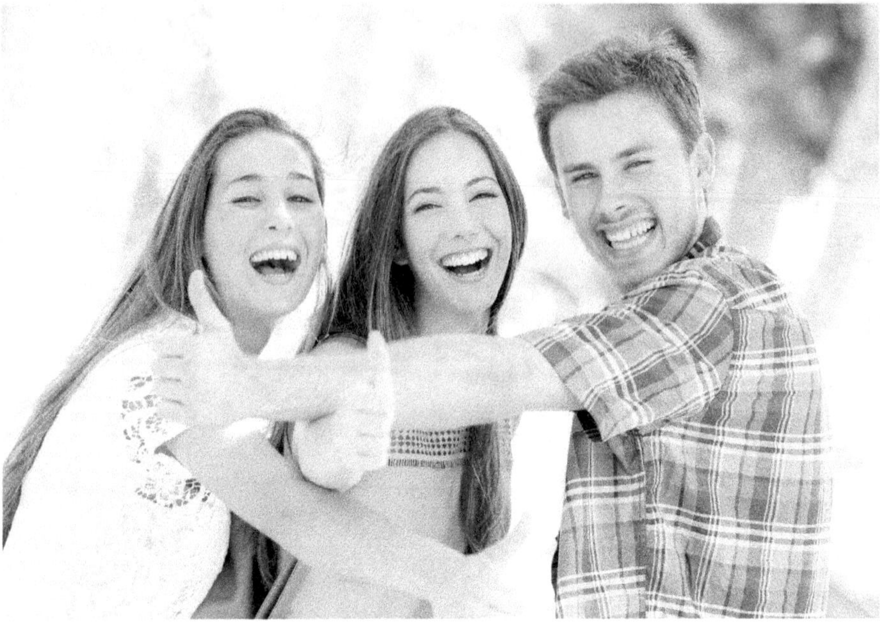

We hope you join us in the 8-week course to learn more about these and other effective steps to lose weight and enhance your energy the natural way!

The Quick and Dirty on Habit Change

"We become what we repeatedly do."

Sean Covey, motivational speaker and author of *The 7 Highly Effective Habits of Teens and The 7 Habits of Happy Kids*

You're about to change something about your eating, and assuming you are at least 3 years old if you are reading this right now, you have already eaten around 3,285 meals! In other words, ***we all have habits around food and eating***. As the above quote illustrates, our actions

---

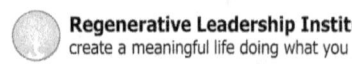

Regenerative Leadership Institute
create a meaningful life doing what you love

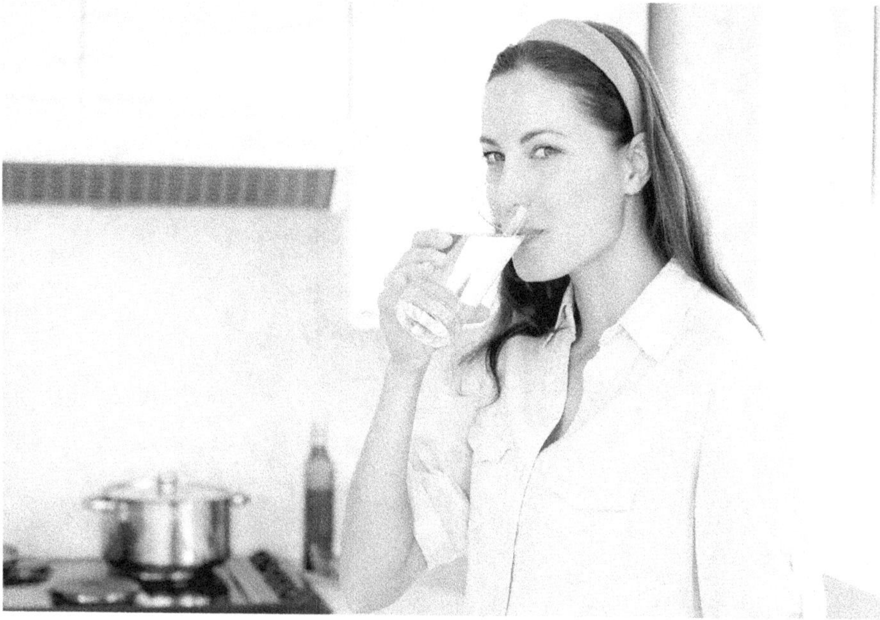

become our habits, and this works in both directions. By intentionally changing and reengineering our actions, we change our habits!

What you need to know about habit change now in order to succeed later:

1. *It's easiest to do what is easiest, so make your new habit as easy as possible to do.*

For example, let's say Chris intends to reduce his intake of highly processed food. He currently has half a bag of cookies left in his cupboard from his nightly I-have-one-cookie-for-dessert-every-night routine. When he signs up for this course and decides to try out this whole food, plant-based thing, he might want to give away those remaining cookies to someone else who wants it. This removes the temptation from his environment, and suddenly makes the desired behavior (ditching the cookies from his diet) the easiest one to perform. This tip has two parts:

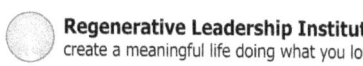

Regenerative Leadership Institute
create a meaningful life doing what you love

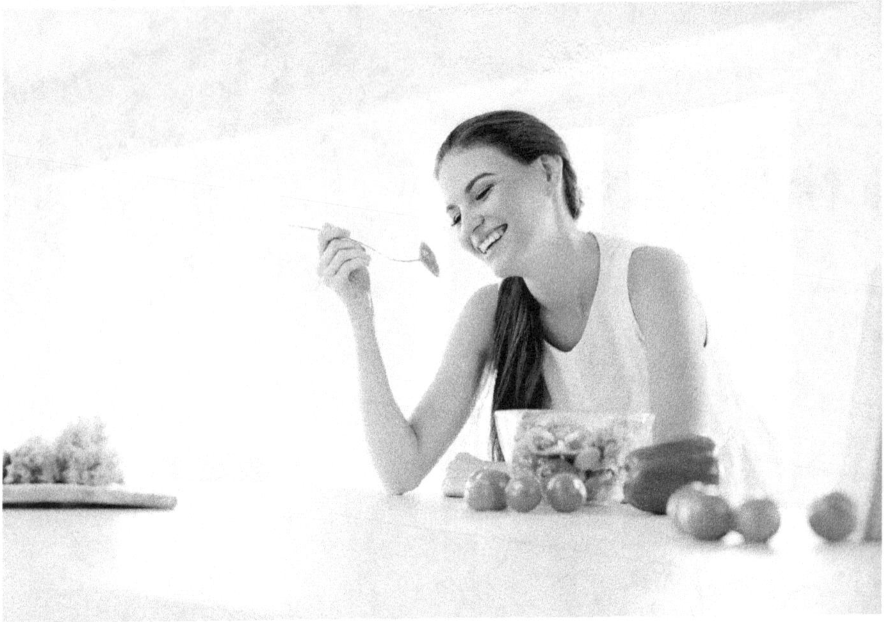

• *Remove temptation to do what you don't want to do.* Get rid of the cookies, Chris!

• *Make it easy to do what you do want to do.* Hey Chris, fill the freezer with frozen fruit so you can enjoy an after-dinner smoothie that helps you ease out of the cookie routine and ease into a much healthier one. Or, take a cue from our sample meal plan and make sure you keep stuffed dates around for your dessert, Chris!

2. *Know the Cue-Routine-Reward cycle.*

Habits are shortcuts in thinking that reduce the number of decisions we have to make throughout the day. We teach ourselves to take a certain path automatically as soon as we recognize we have the option. It's the **Cue** that tells us we are at that choice point. The **Routine** is the path we have taught ourselves to take. The **Reward** is what makes our brains light up in an area called the amygdala. That creates the sensation of pleasure.

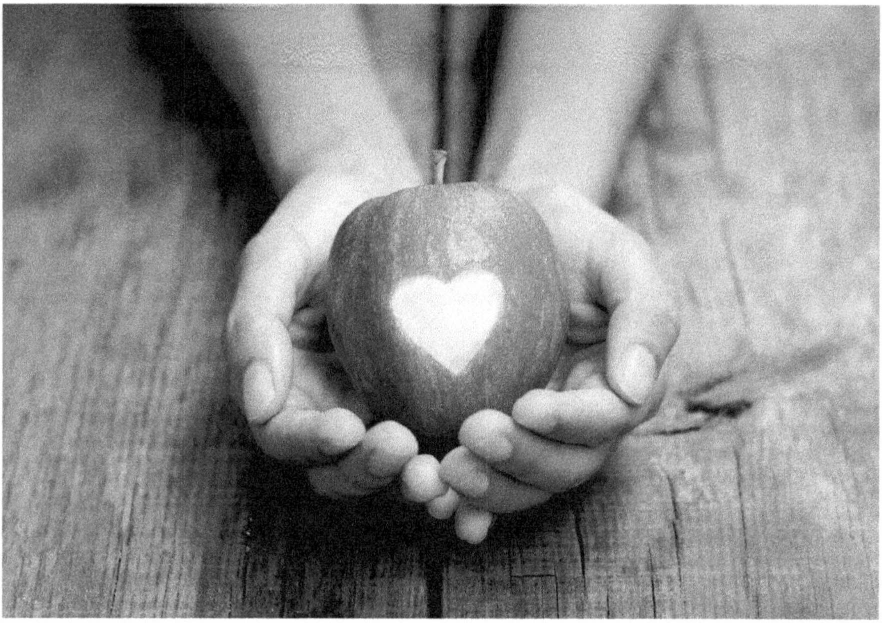

Example: When Pat gets home, she always puts her keys on the table, pours some apple juice, and drinks it while she thumbs through the mail. Then, she starts to feel relaxed and allows her mind to transition from thoughts of work and commuting to her home life.

• ***The Cue:*** Arrive at home

• ***The Routine:*** lay keys on the table, pour juice, and sip while browsing the mail

• ***The Reward:*** Relaxing, calming sensation; the sweet taste of juice; and the anticipation of possibly finding her favorite magazine in the mail.

You can interrupt at the moment of the cue and replace the routine. Pat decides to anticipate the cue and skip the routine. Of course she will arrive at home like any other day, but this time, her new routine will be to drop everything on her bed and take a warm shower first thing when she

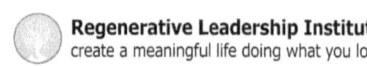

gets in. She is replacing one routine with another for a similar reward - a relaxing, calming sensation and a sense of closure to the work day.

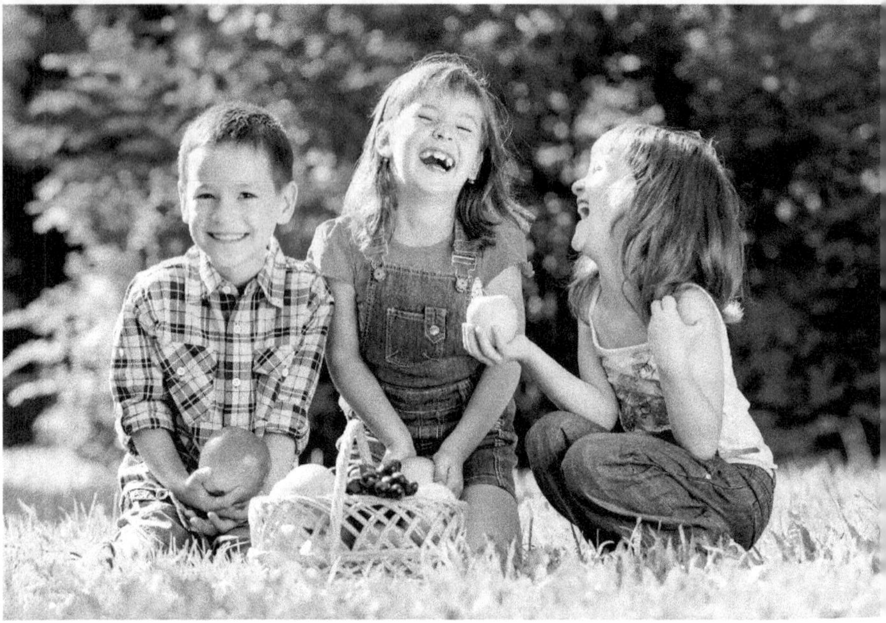

You can tweak the routine. Pat decides to do everything as usual, except that she will replace the large glass of apple juice (no fiber, higher calorie) with a fresh apple (all the juice and sweetness, but also lots of fiber to fill her up on fewer calories and slow the sugar's entry into the bloodstream).

3. External accountability rocks, for some people.
Lots of us will perform way better when we know others are watching. This is true in our work and athletic lives, and it goes for our habits, too. Tell someone about the change you intend to make, and set up an accountability plan with them. Perhaps you check in with them daily or weekly to tell them how it's going. Better yet, find someone who wants to make similar changes and be accountability buddies for each other.

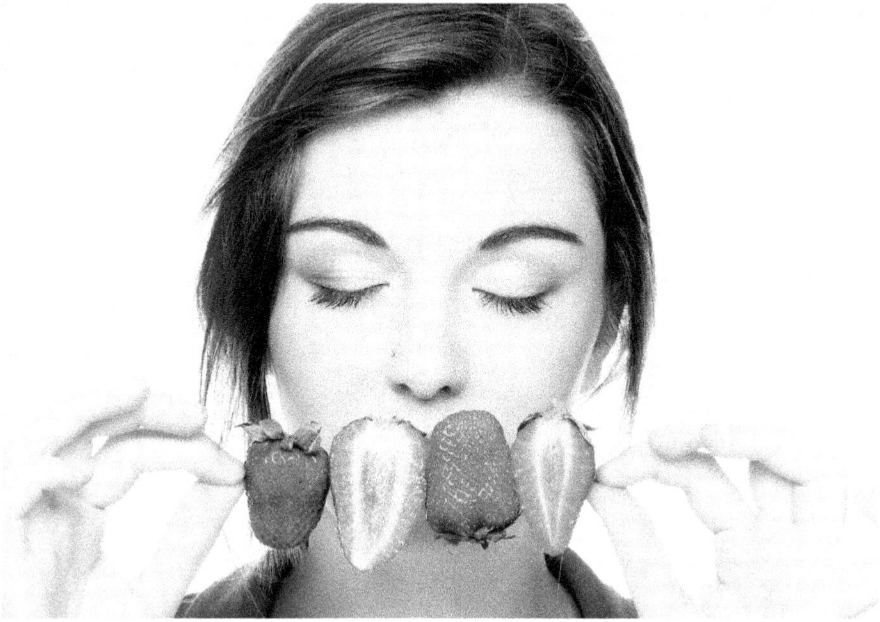

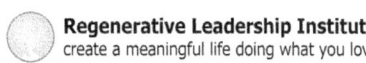

4. Leverage the power of positive reinforcement.

This is commonly known as a reward: You do a good thing, you get a good thing. (We're using "good" and "bad" here for the sake of demonstrating these principles as simply as possible.) For many of us, food is our go-to reward. But you can also use non-edible things to celebrate and reward yourself, and you may eventually find that they nourish you at a deeper, more satisfying level than food does. For example, a massage, a long walk, a book you can't wait to read, a non-cancellable phone or in-person date with a good friend, a trip to an exciting destination, or an extra round of golf this week.

5. Leverage the power of negative reinforcement.

There's a common misconception that negative reinforcement is the same thing as punishment. It isn't. Instead, negative reinforcement means that, if you don't do the desired thing, you don't get a reward. That is, if you don't do a good thing, you don't get a good thing. (Punishment = you do a bad thing, you get a bad thing.) So if you don't eat any vegetables today, you don't get the massage that you could have gotten.

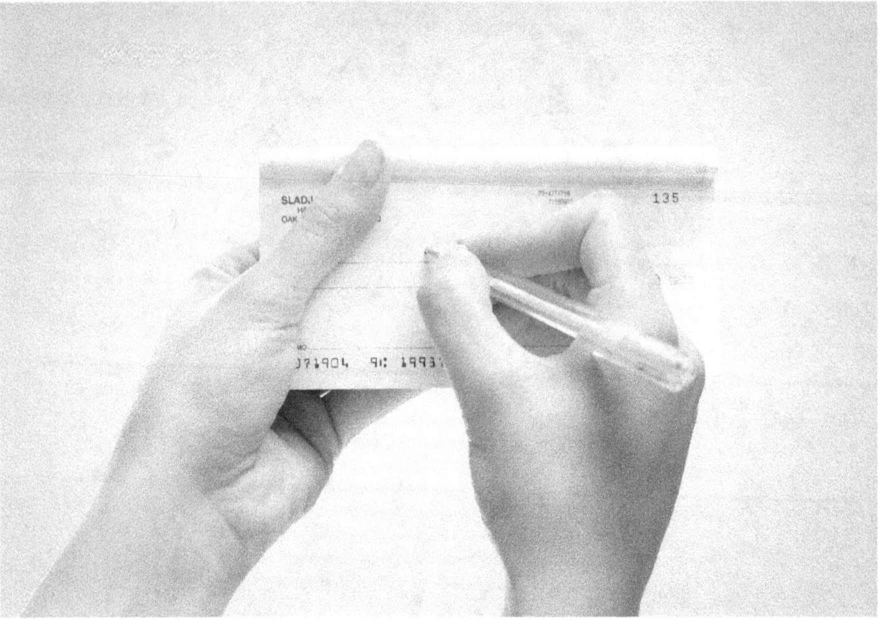

6. Make a bet you can't stand to lose. This last idea is meant to bring a little fun to the idea of external accountability. Here's the idea: Lee wants to make a big change to an old habit. She picks an organization she feels diametrically opposed to. It can be anything as long as she really, *really* wouldn't want to give them a single cent. Ever. Never ever.

Now, she writes a check to that organization for $5 or for $500. (That's how much she disagrees with the organization: she'll do anything not to send that $5!) and asks her buddy Drew to hold it for her. Lee bets that she will exercise for 10 minutes on 4 different days this week. If she doesn't, then Drew will drop the check in the mail come Sunday. If Lee does get her 10 minutes of exercise 4 days this week, then Drew will give her the check and Lee can proudly and gleefully rip it to shreds.

 Regenerative Leadership Institute
create a meaningful life doing what you love

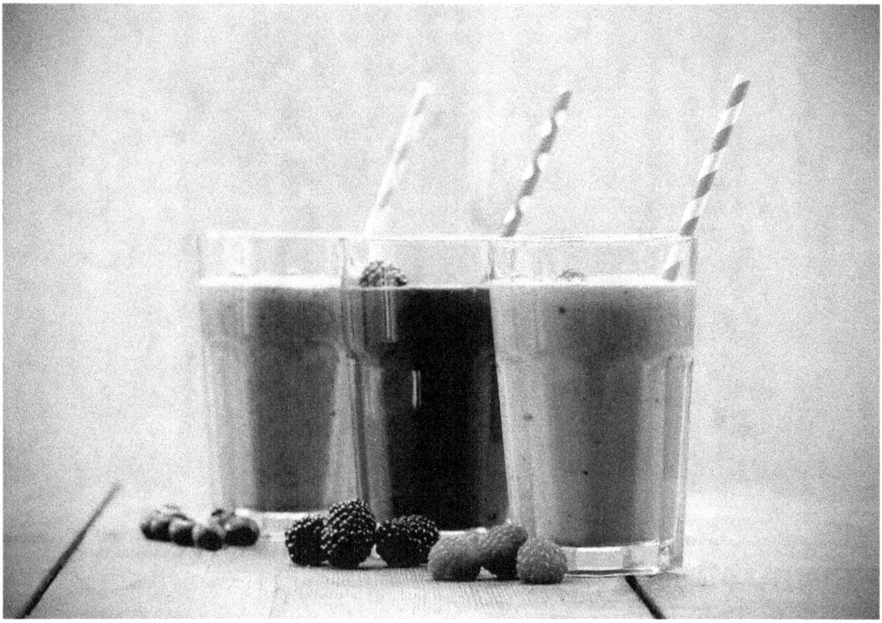

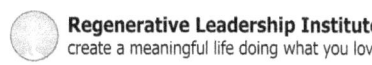

Last Words

"You're off to Great Places! Today is your day! Your mountain is waiting, so... get on your way!"

Dr. Seuss, *Oh, The Places You'll Go!*

You've made it this far. You are ready and committed to creating a healthier life for yourself.

As with so much else in life, you will get out of this what you put into it. The course provides a ton of information, but you are the one who puts it into practice in your own life, and you are the one who determines your success from week to week in the course. In fact, you may have already learned this lesson: when you read this book thoroughly, free from distractions and taking time to reflect on the questions asked, you get more value from the content because you invested more of yourself in the process. If you lightly skimmed this book, skipped over several pages, and/or read it halfheartedly while doing other things, you may have trouble remembering anything from these pages at all, wondering what value you really obtained. In case this happened to you during your first read, start over from the beginning and give it another try – we bet you'll surprise yourself and create something valuable from your experience. Let this book and your participation in the course be the beginning of a powerful story of transformation into the next best version of yourself!

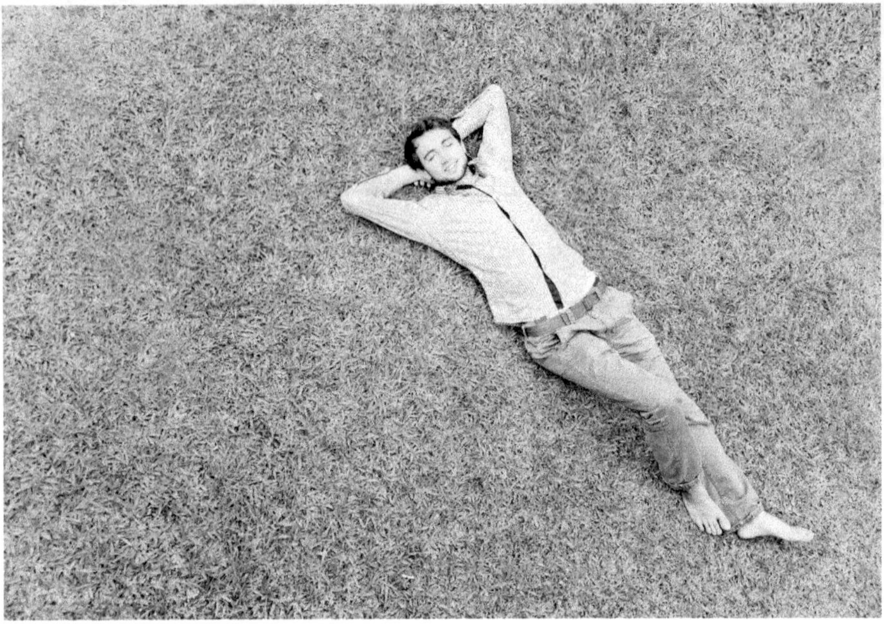

Remember, habit change is a process, and there may be moments when old and familiar habits are pretty tempting. There may even be moments that feel like a step backward. That's all just part of the process. You didn't learn to ride a bike without ever taking a fall. You didn't learn to play an instrument without ever playing one wrong note. Pick yourself back up wherever you are. Start riding again.

More energy, vitality, and well-being await you!

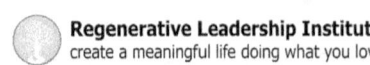

Regenerative Leadership Institute
create a meaningful life doing what you love

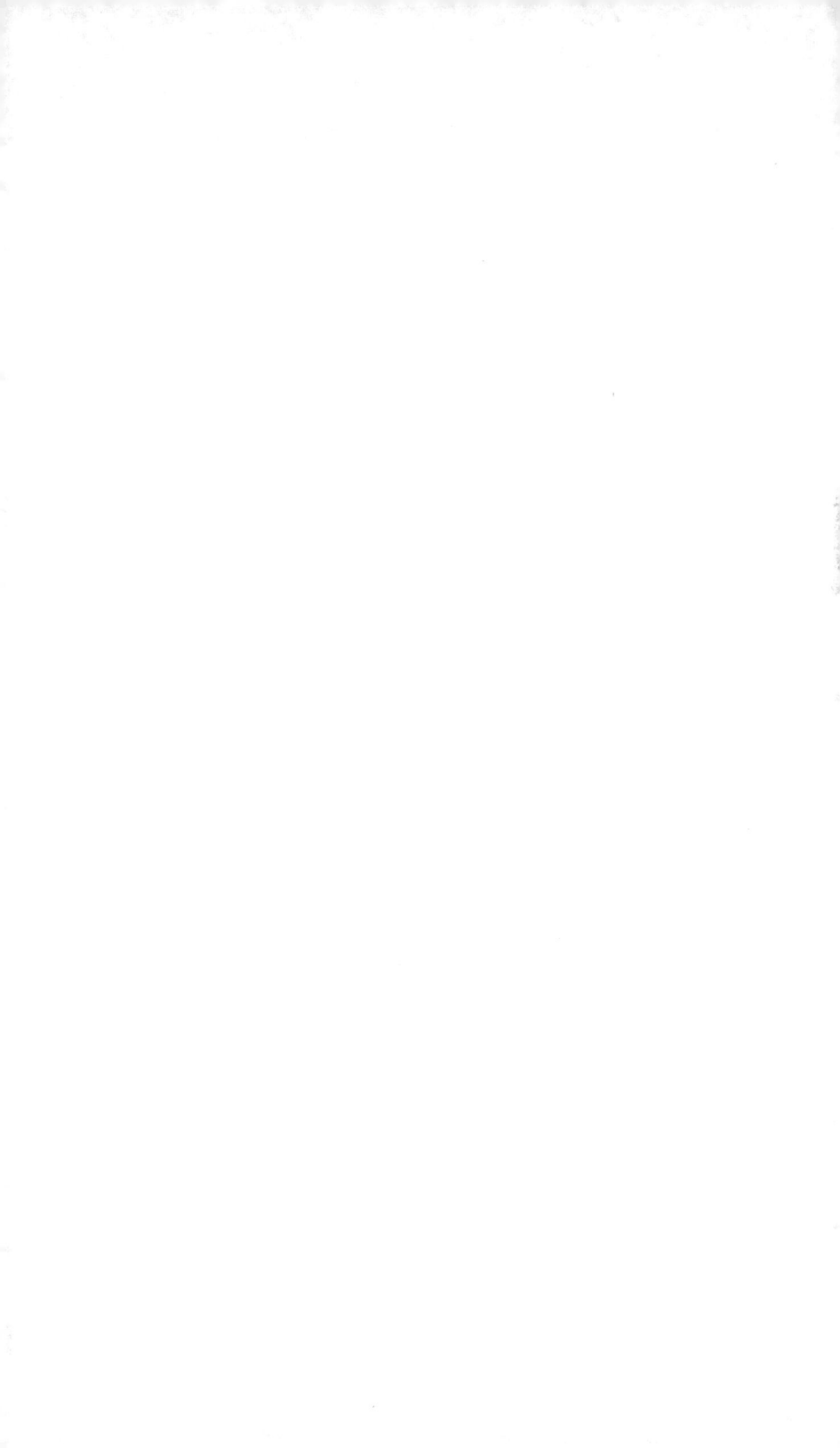

www.ingramcontent.com/pod-product-compliance
Lightning Source LLC
Chambersburg PA
CBHW071325310526
45789CB00016B/921